Praise for Back in Control

"As a society, we want (and need) the specialists who limit their practice to a specific body part or system to treat people as whole people anyway—and to be alert to and provide basic services for problems in other parts or systems. It is IRRESPONSIBLE for any physician (or other healthcare practitioner) to IGNORE symptoms in any domain.

An orthopedist like Dr. Hanscom who is alert to the possibility of psychosocial issues and attends to them is many people's dream of a wonderful doctor."

—Jennifer Christian, M.D.,
Occupational Medicine, President of Webility,
Founder of the Workfitnessdisability Roundtable

"I have been treating patients with chronic pain for over 25 years. Since I have been working with David I have never seen patients experience such a decrease in their pain and improvement in their overall quality of life."

—Suzanne Lacross, PhD.,
Pain Psychologist

"Dr. Hanscom addresses both the prevalent problem of unnecessary spine surgery and the lack of clarity regarding non-operative care. I have the good fortune to work closely with him. His ideas have changed my approach to chronic pain. Our teamwork has given our patients tremendous reassurance knowing that their surgeon and their pain doctor are 'on the same page.'"

—Joel Konikow, M.D.,
Swedish Hospital Pain and Headache Center

"In addition to being a great surgeon, you are a great 'physiatrist.' I appreciate that you look at the person as a whole and address issues of sleep, exercise, and the emotional aspects of pain as opposed to immediately relying on interventional procedures and surgeries."

—Carolyn Marquardt, M.D.,
Physiatrist, Bellevue, WA

"Just learning more about spine surgery and the different options for dealing with pain was very helpful and literally made my back feel better. Dr. Hanscom has a lot of credibility with me because he's undergone back surgery himself and also experienced many of the same things I've struggled with such as anger, victimhood, and anxiety. I am working on these issues and will continue to do so."

—D. I., successful lumbar surgery patient

"I suffered from chronic pain for over ten years but I am currently pain free! It is my hope that others will have the opportunity to benefit from reading this book and that it will dramatically change their lives as well."

—D.H., 68-year-old
with chronic neck pain

"Thank you so much for everything you have done for me over the past four years. You have been the closest thing to a therapist that I have ever had. The DOCC process has treated my ongoing chronic muscle and nerve pain as well as my stress and emotional issues as much or more than the surgery you performed four years ago. You renewed my faith in the medical profession and have given me hope that your concepts will continue to help others and me. I will take all you have taught me and continue to change my life for the better."

—I.L., patient whose persistence over four years
solved her chronic pain

"Hi Dr. Hanscom... the DOCC program seems to have worked for me. My lower back and leg pain have disappeared and I'm a firm believer in the process, especially the concept that anxiety is the driver of tension and pain in many cases."

—K.T., pre-law student who was forced to drop out
of law school due to pain. He is now pursuing pre-med.

"I am grateful that you were my person/surgeon and that you simply cared enough to dig deeper into the healing process and give me the information that I needed at the right time to truly help complete the process... sometimes just giving patients permission to 'be where they are' is healing... especially those of us that manage to put enough pressure on ourselves..."

—T.N., physical therapist who worked for a year to eventually
complete her healingafter a lumbar decompressive surgery

"This book has relevance for anyone with chronic pain, not just those with back/spine or other orthopedic issues. I'd like to see it get a wide readership.

I wanted you to know that your book was very valuable in educating me about what was happening at every stage of my recovery—hence my strong recommendation that you try to reach as many people as possible."

—C.K., reader with a broken shoulder

Back in Control

Back in Control

A spine surgeon's roadmap out of chronic pain

David Hanscom MD

www.back-in-control.com

VERTUS
PRESS

Published by
Vertus Press
3130 East Madison Street #205
Seattle, WA 98112

Publisher's Cataloging-In-Publication Data
(Prepared by The Donohue Group, Inc.)

Hanscom, David.
Back in control : a spine surgeon's roadmap out of chronic pain / David Hanscom.

p. ; cm.

Includes bibliographical references.
ISBN: 978-0-9882729-0-3

1. Backache--Treatment. 2. Chronic pain--Treatment. 3. Chronic pain–Psychological aspects. 4. Mind and body. 5. Spine--Surgery. I. Title.

RD771.B217 H36 2012
617.564/06

First Printing
Printed in the United States of America

Interior Design by GKS Creative
Cover Design by TheDesignOffice.net

While all of the patient stories described in this book are based on true experiences, all of the names are pseudonyms, and some situations have been changed slightly for educational purposes and to protect each individual's privacy.

The information in this book is not offered, nor should it be used to treat or diagnose any particular disease or any particular patient. Neither the author nor the publisher is engaged in rendering professional advice or services to the individual reader.

To my loving wife, Babs,
who supported me through this long journey.
Without her this book would not have been possible.

Disease in man is never exactly the same as disease in an experimental animal, for in man the disease at once affects and is affected by what we call the emotional life. Thus the physician who attempts to take care of the patient while he neglects this factor is as unscientific as the investigator who neglects to control all of the conditions that affect his or her experiment.

...One of the essential qualities of the clinician is interest in humanity, for the secret of care is in caring for the patient.

—Frances Peabody,
The Care of the Patient
JAMA, 1927

Contents

Foreword

For many people, experiencing back pain is like stepping into quicksand. Patients who are otherwise perfectly healthy all of a sudden feel like they're sinking into the depths of pain and despair. They struggle to escape, but just go deeper. Often there was no distinct event or injury that caused the back pain, and so they don't even know how they ended up there.

If their symptoms do not resolve quickly, they do the obvious – confer with their primary care physician. This perfectly logical step too frequently leads to poorly supervised and ineffective care – typically some mixture of medications, physical therapy, spinal manipulation, and various alternative medicine therapies such as acupuncture. If a patient continues to feel pain, his or her primary care physician is likely to recommend consulting with a surgeon.

Many spine surgeons are only too willing to offer help to these patients, who by then are fearful enough and demoralized enough to accept anything that sounds like a solution to their problem. Surgeons rationalize recommending spinal surgery by pointing to a structural abnormality in the patient's spine that is suspected to be the source of the pain. (This rationale can always be given since virtually every adult has deviations from textbook spinal anatomy, even though research has shown that the correlation between spinal pain and many of these "abnormalities" is virtually zero.) The patient undergoes spine surgery, has a poor result, and then embarks on an odyssey to find a practitioner who will give him relief. But instead of relief, there's more pain: they have additional invasive procedures that make their problem worse.

Along the way to this very unfortunate outcome, patients typically develop beliefs and attitudes that seem perfectly sensible, but in fact tend to mire them more deeply in the quicksand, such as:

1. "Since my pain is very severe, there must be something seriously wrong with my spine." This belief embodies the assumption that pain is a result of an injured or diseased body part, and that the severity of pain indicates the severity of the injury/disease.

2. "I have to be very careful about physical activity." When a person has back pain, trivial activities such as sitting in a chair for a few minutes can provoke severe pain. This pain usually leads the person to decrease their overall daily movement, particularly if they suspect that there's been a setback in their recovery. Also, because the patient's pain often started in the absence of any distinct injury, they don't know what might provoke flare-ups in the future, so many people try to "play it safe" by remaining largely sedentary.

3. "Spine surgery is the definitive cure for back pain." Many patients are convinced of this and react angrily when a spine surgeon says that he does not believe that surgery will help. Their reaction is often something like, "If you really knew how badly I hurt, you would offer surgery to me. Since you are advising against surgery, you must not believe me."

As patients search for relief from their back pain, they often operate on the assumption that they can be treated effectively if only they can find the right health care provider. Their reliance on professionals is perfectly understandable – after all, an internet search shows an enormous number of practitioners who tout the effectiveness of their treatments. The advertisements obscure a simple fact though – that for most patients with just spine pain (versus sciatica or arm pain), treatments offered by professionals (including surgeons, nonsurgical physicians, physical therapists, chiropractors, massage therapists, and others) are only modestly effective. In contrast, patients who work collaboratively with practitioners to develop a program of self-directed care can benefit greatly.

This book offers a very welcome approach for patients who are slipping into the quicksand of chronic pain. It provides a complete rundown of conditions and attitudes that interfere with recovery, and gives practical suggestions for strategies patients can use to recover more smoothly and quickly. The ideas in *Back in Control* are not entirely new – other authors have emphasized the importance of practicing self-care to heal back pain. However, Dr. Hanscom has unique insights into the factors that contribute to chronic pain and a unique point of view on the tools that patients can use to extricate themselves from their situation.

Dr. Hanscom discusses the role that emotional dysfunction plays in chronic pain with enormous sensitivity, empathy, and compassion, making for a powerful take on the subject. His approach is truly outstanding, and in my opinion, the book's greatest strength. He points out that patients who become anxious, angry, or depressed about chronic back pain are not "crazy," they are merely reacting normally to very stressful circumstances. He also adroitly uses case histories to flesh out the book's concepts. His vivid descriptions of people he has treated bring the patients to life, making abstract concepts about pain very tangible. The patients' issues and stories are recounted in a respectful manner that in no way diminishes their suffering. As a psychologist as well as a physician specializing in rehabilitation medicine, I wholeheartedly endorse his handling of this topic.

Throughout the book, Dr. Hanscom draws on his personal experiences to outline tools that others with back pain can use in recovery. His personal history, including sciatica and spine surgery, inform his concepts and recommendations; he knows what it is like to be "at the other end of the knife."

He has also confronted his own issues with anxiety, depression, and anger, and has thought deeply about how all three psychological states affected his pain problems. His account of his experience conveys the important message that if a successful spine surgeon and writer can be plagued by emotional demons, it is okay for back pain patients to have them as well.

Another great strength of *Back in Control* is that it doesn't just put forth the issues that plague many chronic pain patients; it provides practical steps that patients can take to dig out of the quicksand. Dr. Hanscom's recommendations are specific enough so that many patients will be able to follow his program without professional help. At the same time, he recognizes the importance of professional help for patients who may need it. Finally, there is a variety of treatments that can be helpful for patients as they deal with the morass of problems that affect the perception of chronic pain. His book presents a framework that organizes these many options in a way that a patient can choose their **own** most effective pathway out of pain based on their own circumstances. This book is not a formula. It just presents concepts, stories, and suggestions. The successful patients are the ones who take care of themselves.

Dr. Hanscom's book contains a wealth of valuable insights for the majority of patients with chronic back pain. Not only is the book insightful but it is also respectful of the suffering that patients with back pain experience. I am eager to recommend it to my back pain patients.

Jim Robinson, MD, Ph.D
Clinical professor, University of Washington Center for Pain Relief

Introduction

When I started my career as an orthopedic spine surgeon in Seattle in 1986, we in the field thought we really had it figured out. Seattle was doing a lot of spine surgery in the late eighties. To provide you with some perspective, we were performing a full nine times the number of procedures per capita as another medical hub, New England. I'd come out of my spine fellowship feeling that surgery was the definitive answer and thinking I could solve almost any spine problem with an operation. I performed dozens of spinal fusions a year for lower back pain. Patients and referring physicians also tend to view surgery as the "final solution," so I felt pressure from all parties to offer it as an option.

Over time, however, I began to see that many of the surgeries were causing more harm than good. Patients often saw little improvement, or none, or they were worse off than before. Some ended up with severe deformities when their spines broke down above and below a fusion. Patients frequently underwent multiple surgeries within a short period of time; I saw some who'd had more than a dozen operations in two years. Much of the time they didn't actually need the initial fusion that led to a cascade of disasters. Surgery *wasn't* solving all spinal problems.

Eventually I came to see that doing fusions for low back pain (LBP) when there is no structural injury (the majority of cases) is the worst thing you can do for a patient. This realization brought me to a major turning point in my career. About seven years into my practice I quit performing fusions for LBP.

Hundreds of thousands of fusions are performed annually in this country for low back pain, most of which I believe are unnecessary. Surgery is a major commitment, so most patients expect their fusion for LBP to solve their pain. It's estimated, however, that this is the outcome in less than a third of cases.

This proliferation of fusions has created a crisis in national orthopedic health care. As an orthopedic surgeon, I am here to say enough false hope. Enough physical damage. Enough unnecessary surgeries.

This is why, in *Back in Control*, I've presented an alternative to surgery, one that dramatically improves function, reduces anxiety, and sets you on the road to a lifetime of better health.

In this book I approach the chronic pain experience differently than most people in the health care industry, especially in its surgical arm. The difference is this: I believe you must address **all** the variables that affect your perception of pain, especially those associated with calming down the nervous system, in order to heal. The term I use for this is comprehensive rehabilitation.

Back in Control reveals the best way to calm a turbo-charged central nervous system and set yourself up for a smooth recovery. In the chronic pain experience, the nervous system is firing on all cylinders, drastically magnifying any pain impulses. These impulses course through the brain and nervous system over and over on a continuous loop. The more pain you experience, the more the impulses are magnified, and vice versa. Eventually these "circuits" are memorized, leading to a vicious circle that can be set off by even the slightest stimulus.

THE DOWNSIDE OF SURGERY

The patients I see with chronic back pain view surgery as the only solution for a condition that has taken over their lives. They are typically physically debilitated and anxiety-ridden. Multiple treatments have often been prescribed, usually in a random fashion, but nothing has worked. In the state of mind patients find themselves in, they're anxious to find a cure—any cure—for their pain. What they aren't aware of, however, is the downside of surgery.

In my twenty-five years as an orthopedic surgeon I've seen thousands of patients who had back surgery—usually a spinal fusion—that didn't meet their expectations. After a painful recovery process their lower back pain was diminished only slightly or not at all. Sometimes there were complications and they had to go back for more surgery. A succession of surgeries may have left them physically and psychologically broken. They regret having had a procedure in the first place and are miserable. A common refrain I hear from patients is, "If I'd known how difficult the surgery would be, I wouldn't have done it." Many of these situations are the result of failed back surgeries that might have been avoided at the outset.

Chronic pain cuts a wide swath. My patients often suffer a great deal, not only from chronic pain but also from the related anxiety and frustration. Their smiles are gone. Their family lives tend to be strained. Family members, instead of serving as a major source of support, are just trying to survive the emotional fallout from their loved one's distress.

I'm grateful to have been given the opportunity to help these patients. However, I'm disturbed by the fact that a significant percentage of their original failed spine surgeries could have been avoided with comprehensive rehabilitation. In spite of my surgeon's bent to perform surgery, the most satisfying part of my practice is directing patients into a structured rehab program that produces consistently good results.

I did not begin my practice with this mindset. In medical school I was taught nothing about chronic pain or comprehensive rehab. I recall a conversation I had with a veteran orthopedic surgeon during my first year of practice. His comment was, "You do a little of this and a little of that, and eventually the pain goes away." What I didn't realize for many years is that it was the *patients* who went away when they became tired of not getting better with such random treatments.

It's well documented in the orthopedic literature that psychosocial stressors like marital problems, difficulty at work, financial issues, etc. are a better predictor of how well a patient will recover from back pain than the specific type of back injury. I didn't understand that idea until I'd been in practice for over ten years. This is why I now give every new patient an extensive spine pain questionnaire that includes many psychosocial questions. I have discovered that, invariably, patients' personal lives, work lives, close relationships, and family support or lack thereof play a major role in their ability to respond well to treatment.

THE DOCC PROGRAM

To treat my chronic pain patients I've developed a system that has helped thousands of them to recover: the DOCC (Defined Organized Comprehensive Care) program.

I started the DOCC program after discovering that by providing a systematic approach to dealing with all aspects of a pain problem, I could almost always help patients become more functional. But more surprising to me was that not only would they become more functional, many would experience a nearly complete recovery. Patients who had been disabled for quite a while would have a remarkable improvement in their pain, come off narcotics, and resume an almost normal lifestyle. Frequently the new lifestyle was more active and satisfying than anything they had experienced before. I had not anticipated that type of response.

If you're in chronic pain, you're usually distraught that you have no control over what is a disabling problem. The DOCC program pulls you out of this desperation by helping you regain control of your health. It takes you step by step through key rehabilitative measures (including improved sleep, stress management, and anxiety reduction) that calm your nervous system and let you take charge. This makes you much better prepared for physical therapy. It also allows you to continue your recovery in an organized, systematic way, overlooking nothing.

Typically, when patients come to see me they've been bounced around the medical industry and their care is completely disorganized. Usually they've had some combination of medication and physical therapy, but there's been no follow-up by the health care system. They're sleep-deprived, anxious, and barely able to function. They're also angry that the medical profession hasn't found a source of their pain and that there's no solution to their severe health problem. You will see as this book progresses that the essence of the problem is that Western medicine has medicalized a neurological disorder.

The DOCC program shifts the focus from searching for the pain source, which may not even be identifiable on a test, to what you can do to become more functional. It addresses all of the factors contributing to chronic pain and a turbo-charged nervous system—lack of sleep, anxiety, medications, goal setting, physical conditioning, and anger—and goes through the best way to deal with them one by one. Each component must be carefully treated to have a successful rehabilitation. Since the medical establishment is not set up to take a comprehensive approach to your care, it's crucial to take your care into your own hands. This program shows how to fill in the gaps left by automatically or randomly assigned treatments and also tells you when to insist on adequate follow-up by your health care providers. It's a much better approach than simply waiting to be told what to do.

In recovery, it's crucial to recognize the connection between pain, anxiety, and frustration. If left unaddressed, the combination of these three factors can create a very dark place in your mind, which I call the "Abyss." It may not be detectable on a psychological test, but it exists on a deep level for every patient suffering from chronic pain.

Part of staying out of the Abyss involves discovering how pain exists in learned neural pathways, similar to the pathways that are laid down when you learn any skill, such as riding a bike or playing the piano. By utilizing certain tools to detach from pain pathways and creating alternative, more functional ones, a patient can calm his or her nervous system. Then, at some point, the pain usually disappears. The major predictor of success is how much (and how well) patients engage in the program over time.

TRAPPED—LABELS, SLEEP, AND STRESS

Chronic pain patients face many challenges: they are often labeled by friends, family, employers, claims examiners, and also physicians as being "unmotivated." Once you're labeled, people can no longer see who you are, much less hear you and try to meet your needs. It's common, if not the rule, for sufferers to become very socially isolated.

This isolation is just one of many stress factors that those in chronic pain must contend with. It's no news that stress affects our health and overall well-being in a major way, but the current medical system has not been set up to help patients deal with stress and it does not reward doctors for the time they spend talking to patients and coordinating their care.

For example, physicians are not routinely trained in the importance of getting enough sleep and/or in how to address this issue. Lack of sleep causes additional stress and inflames your nervous system further, making it difficult if not impossible for healing to take place. The DOCC program shows you how to work with your doctor to make sure you're sleeping eight hours in twenty-four via sleep strategies as well as medication if needed. Outlined in this book are multiple sleep strategies and a complete rundown of sleep medications to educate you about the issue.

In addition to sleep, the program addresses other strategies you can use to manage chronic pain:

- Gain control over anxiety by breaking the cycle of negative thoughts using cognitive behavioral techniques, such as writing and meditation.
- Identify stress-inducing anger issues and become more proactive by giving up victim status and doing cognitive behavioral exercises.
- Understand your medications so you can make better decisions with your doctor about how to optimize them and minimize their side effects.

- Create a vision for how to recover and do goal-setting exercises for living a productive life.

Working along these lines will slow your nervous system so that you can then address your physical pain. If you undertake physical therapy with a fired-up nervous system, any manipulation of your muscles will be excruciating. Once your nervous system isn't blasting on all cylinders, physical therapy will be infinitely more effective. If your system is calm, the muscle work will go smoothly.

The DOCC program will work for any type of orthopedic pain—back, neck, shoulders, elbows, and so on. For the purposes of this book, however, we'll focus on the most common: low back pain.

The program is designed to be implemented in partnership with anyone involved in your care, including your physician, pain psychologist, physiatrist, physical therapist, or chiropractor. Think of it as a team set up to work on each part of your recovery.

You may be thinking, "I've *tried* medication! I've *done* stress management! I *still have pain!*" It's true that you may have already tried one or more of the parts of my program. But it's the step-by-step, structured combination of addressing ALL of the aspects of pain that will make an impact on your quality of life.

By aggressively addressing their sleep issues, setting goals, dealing with any underlying anxiety or anger, and undergoing rehabilitation, my patients have been able to get rid of their chronic pain.

As you recover step by step with the DOCC program, you'll start to lose the feeling of being hopeless and trapped. Instead of letting others make decisions for you, *you'll* be in charge of your own health care.

Throughout, I've included stories of real-life chronic pain patients who've improved their own health dramatically by doing the DOCC program, as well as stories of my own struggles with pain. It's only through firsthand experience—including my journey into extreme anxiety, anger, and victimhood—that I can relate to my patients and help them make it through.

The medical system is not going to change any time soon. The biggest goal of this book is to give you enough information so that you can develop your own resources. To do the DOCC program, it's necessary to be proactive with your health care providers. Not only are physicians not trained in the concept of continuity of care, insurance plans will usually not adequately pay for the resources needed to help you solve your chronic pain. In fact, the medical world is so procedurally oriented that you will usually get moved from treatment to treatment without any continuity at all. Your anxiety and frustration will intensify, which will increase your pain.

As you become more educated about your pain problem and how you can guide your own rehabilitation, however, your anxiety levels will decrease. As you take more control, your anger will diminish. You'll have a significant start on calming down your own nervous system.

If you're frustrated, angry, anxious, and not sleeping, you are simply not in a good place to make a major decision regarding a surgery that will significantly alter your body's anatomy. With the DOCC program, you can get into enough mental and physical shape to step into a new life.

I am not the first person to pose an alternative to back surgery. Indeed, there have been hundreds of books with alternatives: exercise, stress reduction, and the mind-body connection. However, so far no one has looked so closely at the linkage between pain, anxiety, anger, and frustration and conceptualized it in terms of neurological pathways. Treating these factors with the DOCC principles is an extremely effective way to recover from pain—back pain or any other type of pain. It's also the best way to get your life back.

CHAPTER 1

The Path to Chronic Pain

with guest author
Dr. Howard Schubiner

If you're in chronic pain, you're probably wondering how you got to the point where the pain is so debilitating that it's interfering with your life and work. There are an infinite number of circumstances that lead to chronic pain, but some generalizations can be made. Namely, there are four major steps in its evolution:

1. There is a source of the pain, which may or may not be readily identifiable.
2. Your brain becomes sensitized to the pain impulses.
3. Your nervous system memorizes the pain pathways.
4. Sleep, anxiety and anger affect the final perception of pain. I call these three variables the "modifiers."

As a first step in your recovery, it's vital to understand the role these factors are playing in the development of your pain. You must also recognize how you are currently dealing with them.

THE SOURCE OF PAIN: PAIN GENERATOR

I am a surgeon. Like all surgeons, I like to find a source of pain so that I can provide the patient with a solid diagnosis and then fix the problem. When this happens, the patient is happy and I am happy. I'm the hero.

Almost universally, surgeons and patients tend to believe that a structural injury is the source of chronic low back pain, aka the "pain generator." If that injury can be identified and repaired, the thinking goes, the pain will resolve. On the surface, this seems plausible. If you were experiencing intense back pain, you'd think there would be a diagnostic test that could identify its source and point to a solution.

This was one of my guiding principles during my first five years of practice. It was my assumption that if a patient had experienced low back pain for six months, then it was my role to simply find the anatomic source of pain and surgically solve it. I was diligent in this regard.

The test I relied on most heavily was a discogram, where dye is injected into several discs in your lower back. If the injection causes a pain response that's similar to your usual pain, it's considered a positive test. I no longer use the discogram, largely because it's subject to the interpretation of both the physician who is injecting the fluid and the patient. In addition, it has been shown in recent studies not to be a dependable predictor of success when used as a basis for surgery. However, at the time I thought it was the definitive test. If the test came out positive, I would perform a fusion, a procedure in which two or more vertebrae are joined together. I performed dozens of lower back fusions and often felt frustrated when my patients' pain remained about the same. Frequently I couldn't find a way to surgically solve my patients' lower back pain.

Back then, I didn't think in terms of structural versus non-structural sources of pain. Here's the difference: A structural injury is an anatomic abnormality that's distinctly identifiable on a test (such as a ruptured disc or pinched nerve), where the symptoms *match* the location of the abnormality. (For example, if the test shows a pinched nerve and your symptoms don't match—i.e., they aren't present in the area supplied by that nerve, then something's off.) A non-structural injury is generally an injury to the "soft tissues" (muscles or ligaments) supporting the spine. With the soft tissues, the source of the pain is not distinctly identifiable on a diagnostic test, and/or test results come back positive but your symptoms don't match.

In truth, physicians can make an exact diagnosis of the source of lower back pain only about fifteen percent of the time.[1] Generally we do not know the exact cause.

The notion that all pain has an identifiable structural source overlooks several key points: First, soft tissue injury can occur at a level that is below the sensitivity of any diagnostic test. Or tissues can be irritated without being torn—another undetectable injury. The irritation occurs through inflammation, which is a chemical, not a mechanical, issue.

Undetected Injuries

Patients may become frustrated when pain from an "undetectable" injury doesn't let up. They begin to feel that no one believes them. How can a problem with no definitive diagnosis continue to cause so much misery?

If you think this through, though, a soft tissue injury is far more likely to persist than, say, a broken bone. In the spine, once the soft tissues are irritated, they may stay irritated through normal daily activities, sometimes almost indefinitely. If you severely sprained your ankle and kept re-spraining it on a daily basis, how long would it remain painful? On the other hand, broken bones heal in three to four months. The prognosis for a fractured spine has been shown to be better than the prognosis for a muscle sprain.[2]

One of my own muscle/tendon afflictions is tennis elbow. I tend to set it off when I lift a weight that's too heavy at the gym or when I over-practice my terrible golf swing. I will then suffer for months with severe pain in either one or both of my elbows. My two most severe episodes of tennis elbow lasted about eighteen months each. Each one occurred—not coincidentally,

I'm sure—during very stressful periods of my life. During these times, it hurts to shake hands, reach up and adjust the lights during surgery, use the surgical instruments, and do countless other routine activities. The pain is as severe as any pain I have experienced, and it is persistent. Two years after my last bout, I can still push the spot on my elbow and slightly feel the irritated area. Yet if I had an X-ray, MRI, CT scan, or bone scan of the area, the results would be completely negative. If I had a biopsy, there would probably be some inflammatory cells in the tendon area. However, since a biopsy would not change treatment, there would never be a need to do one.

Patients often wonder how soft tissue can be so painful. It's because soft tissues are loaded with small and numerous pain fibers arranged in a kind of spider web pattern. Irritated soft tissues give rise to some of the most painful conditions that afflict us, such as plantar fasciitis, tennis elbow, muscular tension headaches, chondromalacia of the kneecap, and countless more. Even a heart attack is fundamentally a muscular pain: the heart muscle lacks oxygen and the soft tissue pain fibers around it are stimulated. Additionally, emotions can intensify pain. For example, there is a lot of survival anxiety associated with chest pain, especially if there is an actual heart attack occurring. If you are going through an emotional time or there is distress in your life, pain is amplified to a great degree. The pain itself, of course, can also be a great source of distress.

Mind Body Syndrome (MBS)

Over the last year, I was re-introduced to a diagnosis that I'd heard about and written off twenty years ago. It has several names, but the one I was familiar with was "TMS" or "tension myositis syndrome" coined by Dr. John Sarno in his book, *Mind Over Back Pain*.[3] TMS is Dr. Sarno's original term for what we now call "Mind Body Syndrome."

Dr. Sarno, a physical medicine physician, created the diagnosis after seeing thousands of patients with back pain. Upon careful examination and comparison, he found that there was little correlation between their physical examination findings, their X-rays, and how much pain they reported. When he listened closely to their stories, he began to see that emotions (particularly unresolved anger) were typically at the root of their pain. He has written several best-selling books explaining this concept (including *Healing Back Pain*, *The Mindbody Prescription*, and *The Divided Mind*) that have helped thousands of people eliminate chronic back pain. Dr. Sarno hypothesized that unexpressed anger may lead to a constriction of blood vessels that creates pain in tissue structures. Unfortunately, few physicians noticed Dr. Sarno's work, and his revolutionary ideas didn't gain much traction within the medical profession.

I became familiar with an updated view of Dr. Sarno's work when I heard Dr. Howard Schubiner speak about the role of the central nervous system in pain. He is the author of the book *Unlearn Your Pain*,[4] about Mind Body Syndrome. An excellent speaker, Dr. Schubiner turned Seattle on its ear in March of 2011 when he presented the idea that the central nervous system can independently cause pain and other physical symptoms through the development of learned nerve pathways. This is a powerful idea.

I asked Dr. Schubiner to provide feedback on this chapter and explain how he conceptualizes the source of pain in a way that I think is relevant and more complete than the medical world's current view. The next few paragraphs are based on his concepts.

In addition to structural and non-structural injuries, another source of pain is the nervous system itself. When pain is caused by a nerve pathway, there is no tissue damage, there is no lesion; instead, areas of the brain are activated, creating pain and/or causing nerves to fire, which produces tension in muscles or reactions in visceral organs.

Dr. Schubiner divides pain sources into two categories: tissue damage and nerve pathways. The tissue damage category includes structural and non-structural injuries. Categorizing the source of pain would look like this:

Source of Pain
- Tissues
  - Structural
  - Non-structural (not visible)
- Nervous system
  - Mind Body Syndrome—direct triggering of nerve pathways

It's important to remember that in all three of the above scenarios, the nervous system is laying down pain pathways. Although the pathways may be "turned off" at some point, they are permanently imbedded in your brain and can be "woken up" in the future. That's why the central nervous system must be taken into account in every patient every time.

Dr. Schubiner presented recent neurological research demonstrating that the brain has the capacity of neuroplasticity, the ability to create new nerve pathways in response to life events. For example, when you learn to play the piano or swing a golf club, your brain cells are developing new pathways that are connected to your body. These pathways consist of thousands of nerve cells. The more a pathway is activated or practiced, the stronger it becomes. What most doctors do not fully understand is that pain can be *caused* by this type of learned pathway. Even when there's no tissue damage in the body, such as a tumor, a fracture, or an infection, a learned pathway can cause real, physical pain.

In fact, recent research has shown that the brain can create pain that is identical to the pain of a physical injury.[5] We have also learned that an emotional insult is processed in exactly the same way in the brain as a physical insult.[6] We now know that stressful life events and our emotional reactions to them may cause pain that can be severe. Treating this type of pain with pain medications, injections, or surgery is usually not effective, thus leaving the patient extremely frustrated and depressed. However, when the true cause of the pain is recognized, these pathways can be reversed by the DOCC (Defined Organized Comprehensive Care) program.

MBS and Pain

A few years ago, I had a patient named Bill, a middle-aged executive who was experiencing both neck and arm pain. I performed a three-level surgery through the back of his neck to remove bone spurs that were pinching the nerve that runs down the arm. (The surgery was to relieve his arm pain—his neck pain, I felt, was coming from the surrounding soft tissues and therefore couldn't be helped with surgery.) Post-surgery, his arm pain resolved and he wasn't interested in participating in the DOCC program. (Now I discuss pain pathways with every patient and have them do the program, whether they've had surgery or not.) About a year later Bill had a recurrence of symptoms in his arm. His repeat MRI scan showed bone spurs as well as scar tissue that we assumed was causing his pain. I scheduled him for a three-level fusion of his neck, again to relieve his arm pain. This is not a small operation and understandably he was not thrilled to consider another major surgical procedure.

The backdrop to Bill's situation is that he was suffering from severe, unrelenting anxiety and was having an increasingly difficult time in his marriage. He and his wife essentially never talked, which was very upsetting to him.

When Bill came back to me, I'd just heard Dr. Schubiner's lecture and I shared some of his concepts with him. Bill and I talked about how, when prior pain pathways are re-stimulated, the symptoms are essentially the same as the original pain and often of the same intensity. Bill's symptoms were identical to what he'd felt in the past.

Although I did believe that a fusion could potentially help his situation, I also knew it was a very close call, in part because of the difficulty in interpreting an MRI when a patient has had prior surgery. (There is always scar tissue around nerves after any spine surgery and the scan must be interpreted in light of a patient's current symptoms.) Having little to lose, Bill elected to become an active participant in the DOCC program and in the end I did not perform further surgery. Two weeks later his pain was gone and has not returned except for one additional flare-up that was clearly connected to a specific stress in his life and which he took care of on his own. Not only has his pain disappeared, his anxiety has dropped dramatically and he is now coming off of long-term meds for anxiety and depression.

Every week I see patients with neck or back pain (or other symptoms) that are precipitated by stressful life situations and unresolved emotional issues. These experiences have transformed my thinking about many of my patients. I now understand that, often, neurological pathways are either the primary source of pain or are magnifying a prior injury. The gratifying aspect of this for me is that when the actual diagnosis is Mind Body Syndrome, relatively simple treatment through the DOCC program is amazingly effective.

Consider the following scenarios:

Structural Source of Pain
- Surgery successfully solves the structural problem
  - Pain resolved
  - Pain ongoing due to the MBS component
- Surgery does not or cannot solve the problem
  - Ongoing structural source
    ~ Additional MBS component

Soft Tissue Source of Pain
- Surgery is not indicated—ever!!
- Usually treatment cannot be effective with soft tissues until the central nervous system is "calmed down"
  - Still have to consider MBS variable

Mind Body Syndrome
- No identifiable source of pain
- Pain pathways are spontaneously firing

In each of the above scenarios, it's critical to address the pain pathways, which are embedded in your brain. It's similar to riding a bike: once you've learned how to do it, you can't unlearn that skill. You won't think about riding it much during your day-to-day life, but when the bike is in front of you the pathways that allow you to ride it will "wake up."

Addressing the MBS component will decrease pain in all of the situations above except the first one, where surgery successfully relieves the pain. However, even in that scenario MBS concepts may prevent a stress-related recurrence of the symptoms.

My surgical success rate has gone up dramatically in two different ways since I became familiar with the MBS component. I historically have performed many "perfect" surgeries for severe structural problems and been perplexed and frustrated when the pain does not disappear—at all!! I now understand that pain pathways may persistently fire, and this knowledge lets me better help patients with their pain. Now I don't perform *any* surgery (unless it is truly an emergency) unless I can form a partnership with my patient through the DOCC program.

The second impact from learning about MBS is that my "surgical successes" are more successful. Patients don't complain to me as much about how they are "pretty happy with surgery, but..." Their level of residual pain seems to be lower. Additionally, they've experienced a significant decrease in anxiety and frustration and their overall quality of life has improved. Any residual pain has less effect on them.

Summary: The Source of the Pain

Although we often cannot identify the exact structural source of your pain, we do know that the pain centers in your brain are active. The final perception of the pain will depend on how many pain areas are stimulated in the brain. We clearly acknowledge that the patient is not experiencing "imaginary" pain. It doesn't matter why the pain fibers in the brain are firing; they are firing and causing real pain.

If you're one of the unfortunate people who experience pain for longer than a couple of months, your pain may evolve into a *neurological* problem. When the nervous system is barraged day after day with pain impulses, changes occur within the brain itself. As the brain's pain centers remain active they send out signals that alter the body's chemistry. The repetition of the pain impulses and resultant alteration in body chemistry cause you to become sensitized to these signals. Eventually, the central nervous system "memorizes" the pain.

PAIN SENSITIZATION

When the brain is hammered with the same pain impulses day after day, week after week, it becomes more and more efficient in processing them. Subsequently, it takes less of an impulse from your back to elicit the same response in the brain. It's this process that causes patients to complain that their pain is getting much worse in spite of the lack of additional trauma.

This phenomenon was clearly documented in a clinical research study done in 2004.[7] Volunteers who had no significant experience with chronic pain had a carefully measured pressure stimulus applied to their thumb. The response was measured in the brain with a type of MRI that is able to track metabolic activity (called a "functional MRI"). Researchers consistently identified one small area of the brain that responded to the stimulus. They then applied the same stimulus to patients who had experienced chronic pain for more than twelve months. In these patients, *five* parts of the brain lit up. They had a much greater pain response. The difference in intensity of the response was consistent and dramatic.

Water torture provides a crude example of how the brain gets sensitized. In this scenario, a poor prisoner is strapped to a board and water is dripped on his or her forehead. The intensity of drip remains the same, but because of the repetition, the nervous system becomes focused on the dripping and the sensation becomes intolerable. The victim sometimes goes insane. Granted, there are the added elements of fear and of being trapped, but aren't these emotions experienced by those in chronic pain as well?

A less extreme example of pain sensitization took place when a friend of mine, Dennis, was working on a construction site. One day on the job, Dennis placed his hand on the handle of an electric masonry saw which requires a small pump to run water over the blade. At the start of the job in the morning, he felt a very mild tingling sensation when he touched the handle. As the day went on the sensation gradually became stronger. By early afternoon, the tingling was so strong that it felt like an actual shock and he could no longer bring himself to touch the handle.

The two other men on Dennis's crew gave him a hard time at first. They had watched him get more and more cautious, yet when they touched the handle they could barely feel a thing.

The next day they rotated and another guy worked with the saw. Initially he felt only the smallest amount of tingling, just like Dennis, but by mid-afternoon the sensation was so strong that he wouldn't touch the handle either. The third guy now thought they were "playing with him." When he rotated in and first touched the handle, he couldn't feel a thing. But eventually he also wouldn't go near it; he had become a believer. Finally they discovered the culprit: a frayed wire. It was fixed on the fourth day.

What's interesting to me about this story is the degree of the difference in sensation over just six to seven hours of repeated exposure. If the initial sensation from the saw had been strong, the story would have seemed more plausible. However, even though the level of the electric current remained the same, it went from being barely perceptible to feeling like an electric shock. Dennis said that even the anticipation of touching the handle became a problem.

The study, the water torture example, and Dennis's experience demonstrate how the central nervous system becomes more sensitive and the same stimulus recruits more neurons in the brain to fire. In each case, the pain you experience increases with repetition. Of course, you also experience more pain when more actual pain receptors are stimulated—for example, if you get a bad cut or scrape. But whether it's a cut or a sensitized nervous system, the bottom line is that you *feel* the pain. The extent of it depends on the number of neurons firing in your brain. It's quite literally "in your head."

MEMORIZATION OF NEUROLOGICAL CIRCUITS

It is even more fascinating that neurological connections associated with pain will often continue to function even if the offending stimulus is removed. A classic example of this is "phantom limb" pain. It occurs in patients who require an amputation, usually because blood supply to the limb has been compromised by vascular disease. Common causes are diabetes or atherosclerosis, when there's not enough blood to sustain a limb's viability. Prior to the amputation, lack of oxygen causes the limb to become very painful. After the limb is removed, up to 60% of patients feel the pain as though the limb were still there. Almost 40% of sufferers characterize the pain as anywhere from distressing to even *more* severe than before.[8]

There is not a more definitive operation than removing the entire source of pain by performing an amputation. How then do we explain why, post-operation, the patient often feels the same sensations and pain as they did when the limb was attached? This is a dramatic example of the power of the nervous system. It's also a reminder that the brain is an extremely complex, sophisticated computer which is programmable. To "de-program" it takes much more than will power.

An example of a situation where a stimulus was removed but the brain couldn't be "de-programmed" was a major reconstructive spine surgery that I performed in my third year of practice.

Brad, the patient, was a twenty-seven-year-old athletic banker who had a moderate "hunchback" deformity called kyphosis. He was experiencing a lot of pain in the middle of his back. The deformity was about an 80-degree forward curve (the highest normal value is around 55 degrees). I was hesitant to perform surgery, as it would be a major six-hour procedure with significant risks. The surgery went well, however, and his curve was reduced to 50 degrees. However, even though he looked different, his body image didn't change at all, and when his pain did not significantly improve, it became clear that his perception of his looks had been his major issue all along.

I could cite many such examples of negativity. However, the point is that once the nervous system becomes fixated on one specific negative thought pattern, it's not going to stop on its own. The good news is that with specific techniques these circuits can be broken up.

Memorization of Negative Thoughts

In dealing with chronic pain, it's hard not to become demoralized. Months go by, your pain won't go away, and no one seems to know why. You can't help but have negative thoughts, which then become repetitive, just like the repetitive pain signals running through your body. Both are continuous negative sensations to your central nervous system.

The brain becomes so focused on the negative thoughts associated with the pain experience that the thoughts are "memorized," creating new neurological pathways, aka "circuits" in your brain. "The surgeon screwed up my back." "I can't get out of bed." "The pain is ruining my life." These circuits can take on a life of their own, running on a constant loop. If left unchecked, they may turn into a serious obstacle to recovery, one that's not a psychological issue as much as a "programming" issue. (More on this in upcoming chapters.) You become programmed to think the same thoughts over and over again. However, you *can* develop tools to break the cycle of negative thinking, a process

I call "reprogramming." It's much different than the traditional psychological approach to pain.

Feeding Repetitive Thoughts

There are common ways we are taught to deal with repetitive negative thoughts, but most of them are ineffective over the long term. Instead of getting rid of the thoughts, these methods only feed them. Think of these common coping mechanisms in terms of how they affect the neurological pathways in the brain:

1. Suffering
2. Suppressing
3. Masking

Suffering

When you suffer, you have the same set of thoughts over and over, a process that clearly reinforces a given neurological circuit. Suffering takes many forms. Usually it's manifested by complaining, arguing, manipulation, gossiping, etc. There are often strong repetitive thoughts regarding the mess that your life has become. The resulting anger is the jet fuel that gets these circuits really spinning. It's almost impossible to "let it go" because the anger feels so justified. Remember, I haven't even added in the pain.

I recently had a patient who was convinced that somehow the orthopedic surgeon had done a poor job on his rotator cuff surgery five years earlier. He continued to rant about how he'd been irreversibly damaged by this surgeon. (I don't know how well the surgery went versus how well he'd engaged in rehab *after* the surgery.) He was so focused on the story and the sensations around his shoulder that I couldn't even touch his skin around the whole shoulder girdle. Regardless of the reason for his condition, his daily quality of life was additionally compromised by these repetitive, ruminating thoughts.

Note that often patients with chronic pain will see a psychologist for help in dealing with negative thoughts/suffering. This is a generally a good idea—I am a strong proponent of psychological support for almost any situation. However, it must be used in the correct context. In my experience, if your sessions are used only to talk about your problems, you are merely firing up negative neurological circuits and making them more complex. It can be a form of "sophisticated suffering." For psychological interventions to work, you also need a reprogramming component, which we will discuss in Chapter 7.

Worker's Comp and Suffering

Much of the suffering I see in my patients stems from the worker's compensation system. Under worker's comp, your life may have been completely disrupted, your employer may not have treated you very well, and a claims manager has almost complete say over your life. If a worker goes back to light duty they are often harassed. (One steelworker I know who did so was forced to wear a pink hard hat.) Anxiety also becomes a significant issue because there rarely is a clear plan for recovery. These stresses are all in addition to the typical stresses of everyday life.

Suppressing

The second strategy we use to deal with negative thoughts is to suppress them. We don't want to feel negative, so we don't. We think that we have no alternative to a difficult situation, so we put our heads down and just move on.

I have witnessed the downside of this kind of suppression firsthand in the medical profession. In medicine, suppression is a way of life—it's the way we "succeed." We have extreme training conditions, famously long hours, and harsh demands. A law was passed a while ago limiting residents' hours to eighty per week. Those hours are still too many for a given workweek. Think what it must have been like before the law was passed.

Complaining is not an option, though. What can we do? Nothing. So we just put our heads down and go to work. We learn to be "tough." However, the price in terms of mental health is high.

The rate of physician burnout is around 30-40%,[9] and there is a higher prevalence of psychiatric disorders, drug abuse, and alcoholism among physicians compared to the general population.[10] The suicide rate for male physicians is 40% higher than in men in general, and it is 130% higher in women doctors than in their non-medical peers.[11] Four out of eighty of my medical school classmates and two close spine surgeon colleagues committed suicide. The most recent of these was a close friend who was assisting me in two surgery cases. Each case had gone extremely well. Afterward, he shook my hand, said "nice case," and then went out and shot himself three hours later.

Over the years I had watched my friend slowly fold under the stress of being a spine surgeon. He suffered the deadly combination of suppressed anxiety and extreme perfectionism, and burnout was a constant threat. At the time of his death, however, he appeared to have finally gotten a handle on his issues and seemed to be on the right track. None of us saw it coming.

Patients tend to think of their doctors as somehow stronger than they are, and many physicians internalize that projection, not acknowledging even to themselves how much personal damage poorly processed stress is doing to them.

Trying to suppress or not think negative thoughts is a disaster—in my opinion, it may even be more damaging than suffering. The more you try to ignore a negative thought, the stronger it is when it reoccurs. It also takes a significant amount of additional mental and emotional energy to keep such thoughts under wraps.

For example, you might be upset at your spouse, partner, or child because they routinely don't pick up after themselves. The first approach is usually to quietly ask them, which often progresses to nagging, and so on. You also might respond fairly aggressively to effect a change. As you know, neither approach is likely to be successful.

As you are closely connected to this person, you also don't want to be frustrated. So you aren't—you suppress your emotions. When your requests are ignored, you, in turn, try to ignore the untidiness.

Your rational brain kicks in and starts to "keep score." You rationalize that this isn't that big of a deal. There is now a lot of mental energy being expended. You know the rest of the story. The longer you try to ignore the problem, the higher the chance is that you will be irrational when you finally do decide to deal with it.

There has been a movement for decades encouraging people to think positively. In my opinion this philosophy represents a sophisticated form of suppressing. If a situation is bad, it's bad. Pretending otherwise does not help. The energy spent suppressing the negative emotions could be better spent solving the problem. In later chapters, I will offer tools for restructuring your thoughts in order to process any frustrations, such as your family's untidiness, in a more healthy and effective way.

White Bears

In 1987, Dr. Daniel Wegner, a Harvard psychologist, published a paper titled, "The Paradoxical Effects of Thought Suppression." The experiment he devised is commonly referred to as "White Bears."[12] In it, Dr. Wegner divided volunteers into two groups and instructed them to verbalize all their thoughts during a five-minute period in a "stream of consciousness" exercise. During the exercise, they were told either to think or not think of a white bear, depending on which group they were in. Every time they had a "white bear thought" they either rung a bell or verbalized it. This is how it broke down:

- One group was first told to *not* think about white bears for five minutes. Then they were supposed to do the opposite: spend the next five minutes *trying* to think about white bears, all while engaging in the stream of consciousness exercises.
- The other group was instructed initially to think about white bears and then to not think about them during the second five minutes while also continuing the stream of consciousness exercises.

The results were as follows:

- In both groups the participants could diminish the frequency of white bear thoughts when asked to suppress them, but no one could completely get rid of these thoughts.
- In the "expression" part of the experiment (where volunteers were instructed to think about white bears), the number of white bear thoughts increased in both groups.
- In the group who was initially asked to *suppress* the white bear thoughts there was a dramatic increase in the thoughts during the expression phase compared to the group who was asked to think about white bears first.
- The term "rebound" effect was used to describe this large increase. When asked not to think about something, "not thinking" becomes associated with many other cues.
  - The incidence of white bear thoughts actually increased over the five-minute span of expression.

Wegner's experiment shows that trying not to think about something will markedly increase the chances of your thinking about it.

I feel that the insight provided by this experiment is key to the whole mental health aspect of chronic pain. There is a lot of anxiety and extreme frustration that accompanies the chronic pain experience and also a lot of terrible indescribable thoughts, thoughts that are usually so disturbing that we feel we have to suppress them. Well guess what? You are not only fooling yourself by trying to do so, you are also giving these thoughts a lot of power, and over time it eventually takes a tremendous amount of emotional and intellectual energy to ignore them. This is energy you need in order to be creative in solving your problems.

Masking

Masking your reaction to stress is a third way of dealing with repetitive negative thoughts. Masking is behavior that's used to cover up uncomfortable emotions, where you do something to get your mind off of a negative situation. It is usually effective in the short-term, but it is not sustainable. When you're not doing the masking activity, you still have to deal with your racing thoughts. There are several categories of masking, including:

- Addictions
  - Drugs, alcohol, cigarettes
  - Work
  - Sex
  - Gambling
- Getting caught up in a "good cause" (The cause might be excellent, but the driving force behind it could be suspect if examined carefully.)
- Hoarding
- Excessive involvement in hobbies
  - Gardening
  - Reading
  - Sports

Some of the activities listed above, such as hobbies, are not problematic if practiced for the right reasons. If you pursue a deep passion on your own terms and in harmony with your value system, you are creating alternate neurologic pathways that are powerful in improving your mental health. It's an important strategy in neurological reprogramming. However, following your passion is a completely different process than being driven by anxiety. It's impossible to outrun your anxiety without paying some price.

Masking strategies, even when anxiety-driven, might be slightly more effective than suffering or suppressing in that they are not directly feeding the negative circuits. They are not slowing them down, either, though. When you are done with that particular activity, the repetitive negative thoughts are still there. What's more, if you are involved in some type of chemical addiction, there are often physical consequences.

Suffering, Suppressing, Masking, and Pain

Now let's put pain back into picture. The first two strategies—suffering and suppressing—clearly don't work. If you are openly suffering with your pain, over time the pain circuits will be reinforced. If you're trying to suppress, it's almost impossible not to think of your pain for any sustained length of time and those repressed circuits will grow to be monsters. Masking the pain with one of the above choices might work for a small amount of time, but the pain will still be there after the masking activity is over. You will continue to become more and more angry and frustrated. Pretty soon many patients don't have the energy to distract themselves even for short periods of time. The pain consumes their whole life.

Stop reading just for a few minutes and really try to understand and internalize how you personally utilize the three strategies of suffering, suppressing, and masking. All of us do. These are the only methods that I was ever taught. Suffering may come naturally, or you might've been taught to just buck up and be strong. Similarly, you may have been taught to suppress whatever makes you uncomfortable. And certainly society feeds off creating ways to mask stress. But stop and think how these methods may be preventing you from having a deep, connected, joyous quality of life. We'll talk about more healthy ways to break patterns of negative thought in the upcoming chapters.

THE MODIFIERS: SLEEP, ANXIETY, AND ANGER

To review, we've discussed that either there is first an anatomic/physiologic injury that initiates a pain impulse, or the pain impulse occurs spontaneously (MBS). When you feel this pain over a period of time, the nervous system becomes sensitized to the pain impulses. Eventually your nervous system will memorize part or all of the pain circuits.

This sequence is intertwined with another series of events I've called the modifiers. The modifiers are the sum of the emotional response to chronic pain. Patients often become anxious, frustrated, and angry; they lose sleep and their stress levels rise.

Pain modifiers are important to understand because under stress your body chemistry changes. Your stress hormones, including cortisol and adrenaline, become elevated. Adrenaline is the "fight or flight" hormone; when secreted, it causes your heart to race, your blood pressure to go up, and your mind to experience anxiety. Cortisol has more of a chronic effect. It keeps your body hyped up to deal with physical stress.

As a result, several things happen. Your pain receptors and nervous system now exist in a different chemical environment, even though there's no additional physical affliction, or perhaps no physical affliction to begin with. What's the ultimate result? Your senses are heightened and you may experience even more pain.

In addition, your decision-making skills are affected: that's why it's crucial to address the emotional aspect of pain before deciding whether to get surgery.

The modifiers that we'll discuss are sleep, anxiety, and anger.

Sleep

Incorporating sleep into my treatment of pain was my first step in conceiving the DOCC program. I felt I had a whole new weapon that was very effective and simple. Once I was successful in getting my patients to sleep better, there was always some improvement in their sense of well-being if not also in their pain.

Most patients with chronic pain sleep poorly and are tired during daylight hours. They often feel pain more keenly at night, when they have fewer distractions, and a good night's sleep is difficult to attain. But without adequate sleep, quality of life is compromised and day-to-day stress and pain are difficult to handle. Perception of pain is altered.

I started to incorporate sleep treatment into my practice around 1997. If a patient had an acute problem such as a ruptured disc, I would use sleep medications in addition to any pain medications. It was much easier for my patients to make it through the healing process if they were able to sleep well. Whenever chronic pain was involved, the results were the same: with consistent sleep, a patient's mood and coping mechanisms would improve over two to four weeks. If they could not get enough sleep, I would aggressively keep switching meds until we found the right treatment. Not sleeping was not an option.

The first step in the DOCC program is to get at least a month of adequate sleep. It is an integral part of calming down the nervous system. None of the other elements of the program will be effective unless you are rested. Many adults think they can get by on less than eight hours of sleep, but consider it a minimum. Most people, especially if they have chronic pain, do not experience a full night's sleep consistently.

There was one study done in which female volunteers were measured in terms of the quality of their Stage V sleep, also called REM sleep, for a period of time. This is the stage where the most dreaming takes place. It was discovered that the less amount (and poorer quality) a subject's REM sleep, the higher her sensitivity to pain.[13]

I had one fifty-year-old businessman who had experienced chronic neck pain for almost two years. There was no specific injury. He continued to work as an owner of a small accounting firm but was miserable. Extensive physical therapy had been no help. I started a strong sleep medication, which immediately allowed him to sleep a full night. After two weeks, the medication was still working well and the plan was to start him on an aggressive physical therapy program. However, by his eight-week visit I was surprised to find he was completely pain free. The power of sleep had never been so apparent.

Again, my first obligation is to simply get my patients to sleep well. Patients argue with me that it's impossible to sleep with the pain. There are very few situations, though, where the right combination of medications won't yield a consistent good night's sleep in spite of the pain.

Anxiety

A significant part of human existence revolves around avoiding or reducing anxiety. The ability to deal with anxiety in a healthy way is critical to quality of life. It's even more important for someone who experiences chronic pain.

There are several principles I have learned from my own experience and from working with my patients:

- Anxiety is both normal and necessary—it will never disappear. It helps us to identify situations that would potentially endanger our survival, which every human is programmed to avoid.
- It's important to identify both the sources of your anxiety and your reaction to anxiety.
- Untreated, disruptive anxiety always gets worse. It will NEVER get better on its own.
- The more you try to suppress fear, the stronger it will become.
- Avoiding anxiety becomes its own stressor.
- It's necessary to become comfortable with anxiety.
- Anxiety is highly treatable: if it's acknowledged and treated properly, there is a strong chance it will decrease sharply.

I did not become a major spinal deformity surgeon by experiencing anxiety; I succeeded by suppressing it until I was in my thirties. Until that point, I never allowed myself to feel anxious—I was always just a doer and plowed ahead regardless of any adversity. Not succeeding was not an option. I think the reason I suppressed anxiety so well for so long was that I was always in control. Control is probably one of the most effective and common strategies for dealing with anxiety. However, it's also not conducive to rich and rewarding relationships.

I did not start facing up to my anxiety until I started to have physical manifestations that I could no longer avoid. My first hint that it was an issue was one I could only see in retrospect. In 1988 I started to sweat during surgery, which turned into a regular occurrence. I couldn't understand why it happened; it had never been an issue in my training.

Then, a year later, I started to have a little trouble with sleep; I noticed that my heart would race when I tried to fall asleep at night. I felt a little wired but I was still not putting the picture together.

Finally, while driving across a bridge in 1991, I experienced a panic attack. It was about ten o'clock at night in the middle of a driving rainstorm and I thought I was going to pass out and run off the road. My pulse was racing and I broke out in a cold sweat. I had no idea what was going on—I thought I was going to die. It was the first of many such attacks.

By 1997 I had progressed to a full-blown obsessive-compulsive disorder (OCD), which is the ultimate anxiety disorder. OCD is manifested by intense, anxiety-producing, "intrusive" thoughts. However I never had any of the most common outward manifestations of this disorder, such as hand washing. Instead, I had what's called "internal OCD." With internal OCD, you have intrusive thoughts that are countered by "counter-thoughts." The more I fought these thoughts, the worse they became. Needless to say, the process took up a lot of my emotional energy. I did not pull out of it until 2003.

Up until the anxiety started to increase, I had been able to control enough of my external environment that I really didn't experience much of it, and so it was extremely humbling when my body "rebelled" with anxiety-related reactions. You can't control a bodily function such as sweating, racing heartbeat, etc. For the first time, I was not "in control."

It's critical to understand and acknowledge your own anxiety. Being a high-level surgeon, I had refused for many years to acknowledge that it could exist within me. But anxiety is a universal part of the human experience. In fact, from an evolutionary standpoint, the species that were the most hyper-vigilant were the most likely ones to live the longest and to produce offspring. Your anxiety is well founded in the survival instinct.

Uncontrolled anxiety, however, will alter your perception of pain and your ability to cope with it. I find it tragic that such a treatable problem is often not adequately addressed. Methods for coping with anxiety are provided in later chapters.

Anger

Anger is as important as anxiety when it comes to chronic pain management. Some people are able to come to grips with anger and process it in healthy ways. For others, anger erodes their quality of life. Forget about physical pain for a moment. Instead, visualize a day when you were angry with a relative, co-worker, or a troubling situation. What was your quality of life like that day? Not great, right? When you add in physical pain, the day can become intolerable.

In this way, a treacherous cycle forms. You experience chronic pain in addition to the rest of your life stresses. The pain produces anxiety because you don't know where it's coming from and you don't get adequate answers from your doctor. Over time, you become angry about the pain, the lack of answers, the dashed hopes, and your loss of control. As your nervous system gets more and more fired up, your pain increases—and in turn feeds back into the cycle.

Anger is an understandable response to chronic pain, and in my experience, the more legitimate your anger, the harder it is to let go.

But anger, no matter how legitimate, will destroy you and your quality of life. I will cover how best to deal with anger management later in the book. Here, I will share several stories to illustrate how coping with anger in a constructive way can help calm the nervous system and physically decrease your pain.

My own experience with chronic pain helped me to understand the central role that anger plays in it, and the way I eventually broke away from it informed my creation of the DOCC program.

When I was a resident at the University of Hawaii in the early eighties, I noticed that when I went out for a run, the soles of my feet would burn. I blamed it on the warm pavement. However, the feeling persisted after I moved to the mainland, and I realized that I had some type of peripheral neuropathy. In other words, the very small sensory nerves in my feet were firing spontaneously. For years, the warm feeling on my soles was annoying but not particularly painful and it did not in any way limit my activities.

My foot issue remained merely a minor annoyance until much later, in 1998, when I was going through a divorce. It was a difficult time, and I had not yet learned many of the stress management techniques presented in this book. One night when I was sitting in my car, feeling extremely frustrated at the thought that my family would be breaking up, I began to feel a warm sensation in both feet. Within eight hours, it had escalated to a severe burning pain. No matter what I did it would not abate. It interfered with every aspect of my life, including my clinic obligations. I could concentrate during surgery but would have to stop every fifteen minutes or so to refocus. It was even worse when I was relaxed because there were no distractions. I became increasingly frustrated and despondent.

I asked my colleagues for help, and the conclusion was that I had an untreatable heredity polyneuropathy. I was placed on Neurontin, an anti-seizure drug, which had no effect. I couldn't take narcotics because I was actively performing spine surgery. I became quite depressed and was extremely angry about the diminished quality of life that stemmed from my chronic foot pain. I had also lost most of my assets during this time.

I had historically dealt with anger through denial—I simply refused to become angry. However, the intensity and persistence of the pain in my feet broke through the denial and I became extremely angry. This started in January of 2001 and was still in full gear by summer. I woke up angry every morning.

I had instructed my patients that it was deadly to hold on to anger, and now it was me who could not let it go. Intellectually I believed I had done so, but my actions showed otherwise. Anger was like a cancer chewing me up.

There I was, not only angry but also depressed and feeling sorry for myself about being depressed. The self-pity was even more unpleasant than feeling down. Finally, after many months of this ordeal, I came to realize that I was a victim of my own depression. Somehow this realization allowed me to dig into my situation more deeply and begin to move forward. I decided that I was done playing the victim.

I started by going through a very difficult self-examination process. One crucial step was to turn to cognitive behavioral therapy (CBT) via the book *Feeling Good* by David Burns.[14] Burns's first plea to readers was to write about their lives, so I began to write. I could not stop writing. In retrospect, the writing is what pulled me out of my tailspin.

I had always told my patients that if they dealt with anxiety and anger in a pro-active way the pain would not necessarily dissipate, but they would be able to more easily tolerate it. The surprise and shock to me was that in the months that followed my decision not to be a victim, my pain began to decrease; by January of 2003, I was back to where I'd been before the flare-up started. Today, my pain persists, but only at the level it was when it first started twenty-four years ago. This transformation was not a matter of enduring the pain, mind over matter, positive thinking, or using medications; I was able to reduce my suffering by letting go of anger.

Another story about how anger can affect the perception of pain involves one of my patients who had a complication from a revision spine fusion. Mike was a fifty-two-year-old respiratory therapist who was very active, up to the point of running marathons. Many years after an initial spine fusion at L5-S1 at age thirty, his spine broke down above the level of the prior fusion and became very unstable. He waited almost five years before talking to a surgeon.

I performed surgery through Mike's abdomen to place a hollow cage filled with bone graft at L4-5, the level just above his prior fusion. The purpose of the cage was to stabilize the spine as well as to improve the chances of a successful fusion. Still under anesthesia, he was turned over and had screws placed into the vertebrae to further increase the likelihood of a good outcome.

The surgery went very well and Mike felt much better for a few weeks, good enough, in fact, that he increased his activity too quickly, which placed too much stress on the screws. For reasons that were unclear, he also had very soft bone. The screws broke out of the bone and irritated the fifth nerve root that travels down the side of the leg. His sciatic pain was unbearable.

I took Mike back to surgery to re-do the placement of the screws. Post-surgery, his nerve, already irritated and painful, did not calm down and he developed continuous, severe, burning leg pain.

At his one-month check-up, Mike exploded at me. His hour-long rant was not rational. Nothing I could say calmed him down. Afterward, he apologized. He said he was angry at the situation, not at me.

I was not in a great state of mind after his verbal barrage, but elected to hang in there with him and began to apply the DOCC principles. Mike's pain improved with aggressive pain medications. We also aggressively addressed a long-term problem with sleep. After some initial resistance, he engaged in the exercises in the *Feeling Good* book and started to look at his pain from a stress management point of view. He began to consistently write down his disruptive thoughts and then write down more rational ones.

At about three months after the second operation Mike's nervous system had calmed down enough to do aggressive physical therapy. (If you do physical therapy too early, while the nervous system is still fired up, it just ignites the pain and backfires.) About six months into the healing process, he was doing much better. He had calmed down, and so had his leg pain.

Mike's rehabilitation was difficult. He would be doing extremely well with little or no pain and then suddenly have severe flare-ups. At first it wasn't clear what was causing this back-and-forth. Gradually, however, he came see the link between his stress levels and his pain.

About six months into his recovery Mike went back to his job. In spite of the work he'd already done, he was still asked by his employer to participate in a month-long anger management class, which had an additional and dramatic impact on his ability to process his anger.

One year after the surgeries, the program had worked—Mike's chronic pain was gone. He sometimes had a slight twinge, but only when he became frustrated; it was nothing like the severe pain he had felt before his surgeries. At his two-year follow-up, he was back to work full time and had improved to the point where he was running marathons again. In addition to solving his back problems, he was able to enjoy his relationships and his life. As painful (in all senses of that word) as the experience was for both my patient and me, his journey was a gift to both of us.

Acknowledging Your Anger/Victim Status

Every patient with chronic pain I have ever met is angry. You cannot experience ongoing, disabling chronic pain and *not* be angry—it's not humanly possible. However, many patients don't acknowledge their anger to me or even to themselves, at least initially. The ability to hide your anger from yourself is astounding. I often have patients who insist that life is otherwise great except for their chronic pain. Their underlying anger is apparent, but they cover it up, insisting "everything is fine." They'll make comments about "the doctor that did the wrong operation" or wonder, "How could I have undergone so many operations that haven't worked?" They may have lost their job and/or gotten bounced around the health care system, and they are experiencing significant lifestyle limitations. It's more than enough to make anyone angry. The emotional tension is clear to me, but often they really cannot see it. They also don't want to engage in any self-discovery process. The elephant in the room is their chronic pain, disability, and general unhappiness.

My personal metaphor for holding in anger is building a nuclear waste dump. There is a core of very dangerous material that has to be deeply buried under a layer of thick protective covering. It takes a lot of a person's life energy to keep all that material so far down inside. When I hit my core anger in 2003, it was like an oil well blowing off. It was as unpleasant an experience as I could imagine. It did not feel good or cathartic in the least; it felt dirty, ugly, and despicable. However, I now have much more energy to live my life than I had even in high school. That experience changed my life.

If you are dealing with your own anger, my hope is that you can acknowledge it, deal with it, and let it go. You cannot move forward until you connect with what's going on inside of you. It's a vital part of getting better.

Depression and Chronic Pain

You may have wondered why I have mentioned depression as it relates to chronic pain only in passing. There is undoubtedly a strong link between the two. However, I believe that depression in the chronic pain setting is often the result of pain, lack of sleep, and prolonged anxiety and anger. In my experience, treatment of these other problems will resolve the depression. If it doesn't, it's best to consult a psychologist or psychiatrist.

THE PATH TO CHRONIC PAIN: A SUMMARY

The source of your pain may be an identifiable structural anatomic problem or it may stem from chronic inflammation of the soft tissues around the spine. It can also be a manifestation of the Mind Body Syndrome. It is your physician's responsibility to identify the difference.

Once the structural issues have been either ruled out or treated, you're left with the soft tissues and/or the central nervous system. Remember that while pain is never imaginary or "merely psychological," its severity is determined by how your brain experiences it. If the nervous system is subjected to repetitive negative impulses, it becomes sensitized to them. This is true for both pain and repetitive negative thoughts. Eventually neurological pathways are created which have memorized these negative circuits. The pain is intensified. Finally, the situation is made much worse by lack of sleep, anxiety, and anger.

If your central nervous system is "on fire" you will not be able to tolerate manipulation of these already inflamed tissues in physical therapy; your brain will experience an exaggerated response. The next step, therefore, is to calm down the nervous system by addressing the factors that rev it up.

CHAPTER 2

Reversing the Chronic Pain Process

Once you understand how you came to experience chronic back pain, it's time to start pulling yourself out of it. You can do this by gaining an understanding of your problem and learning the related "language" in order to move forward on your own terms. It's crucial to take action and work with your doctor instead of waiting for all the answers from the medical system. That's where the DOCC (Defined, Organized, Comprehensive Care) program comes in.

DOCC is a way of organizing your care so that you have an overall plan and a framework for carrying out that plan. Following the program will build confidence by making you feel more in control and less anxious. Instead of being at the mercy of your circumstances, you can take charge of them. Throughout all of this, remember the distinction that needs to be made between chronic pain and disability: disability may result from chronic pain, but not all people with chronic pain are disabled by it.

DIAGNOSIS

The first phase of the DOCC program is to consider whether the source of your back pain is structural or non-structural. To figure this out, work in concert with your doctor. My goal is to provide you with enough information so you can engage in an in-depth conversation about your specific anatomic problem.

Once you've labeled your problem as structural or non-structural, you can decide on surgery. (Structural problems typically require surgery; non-structural do not.) This decision needs to be made, and very clear in your mind, before you start the DOCC program. As long as any question exists for you, it will be difficult if not impossible to be fully committed.

In my practice, if a patient's problem is structural and significant, I will move ahead with surgery relatively quickly and implement the DOCC program later. If the problem is structural but not severe, then we may attempt the program to see if there's enough of an improvement to avoid surgery.

If the problem is *not* structural, then the only other possible source of the pain is an injury to the soft tissues around the spine. This is the most important distinction I make as an orthopedic surgeon. With non-structural issues, I do not recommend surgery under any circumstances. I spend a significant percentage of my time in my practice not only telling my patients that they don't need surgery, but also explaining *why* they don't need it. This is a critical part of my job and it clarifies the situation for the rehabilitation doctors I work with, so the whole team can move forward in sync.

It's also important to consider the diagnosis of Mind Body Syndrome described in Chapter 1. In this scenario, you may have recovered physically from a structural or non-structural injury, but your brain, when triggered by certain emotions, traumatic events, or other stimuli, can reproduce the painful physical symptoms you felt when you were first injured. Or, you may never have had a specific injury, but your unresolved emotions are triggering pain. MBS can be treated with the DOCC program using methods such as creating alternative neurological circuits. I've been surprised at the array of different symptoms that will disappear with proper treatment.

If one of my patients needs to hear this message from some-one else, I strongly encourage him or her to get a second opinion. If I feel the second opinion is way off, I don't hesitate to call the other surgeon to ask for clarification, and if a case is controversial, I'll also present it to colleagues for feedback.

Remember that by virtue of having lived in misery with pain for a long time, you'll be vulnerable to a surgeon walking into the room and saying, "I can take care of you with surgery." Surgery is viewed by almost everyone as "definitive." How can you turn it down? However, you may be undergoing an operation that is not only unnecessary but also potentially damaging, one that can negatively affect your quality of life permanently. Do not trust anyone, including me, to tell you what to do. Research your problem with a vengeance so that you fully understand your own situation.

It can sometimes be difficult for patients to accept that their problem is, essentially, "undetectable." They are in so much pain that it seems impossible that so many tests would come up negative.

I had one forty-something patient, Gina, who was having a tough time with ongoing low back pain (in addition to some right leg pain), and was understandably anxious about her diag-nosis. She'd been injured at her waitressing job a year and a half earlier: reaching across a table, she'd felt a pop in her back. Gina had been in the worker's compensation system for over a year and had experienced the usual frustration of not being able to work, not getting medical clearance, and having ongoing severe, unrelenting LBP. To add insult to injury, they closed her claim and she ended up losing her house. She was also trying to care for her young child. By the time she saw me, she was in a lot of pain and very unhappy.

I re-opened Gina's claim and then did every diagnostic test possible to identify the source of her pain. All of her tests were completely negative, so I concluded that she must have a non-structural problem. I started her on the DOCC program and she became somewhat engaged, but was not progressing as well as I thought she should. I sensed she was holding back, so finally I sat down with her and said, "Look, what's going on?" She exploded. She was positive that I was missing something structural. I explained to her that this was possible but unlikely, given the degree of testing we'd already done. She remained unconvinced, though, and it quickly became clear that she was not going to let this one go. So she fired me. In the end, her attachment to finding a structural source of her pain was hindering her chances of recovery. Unfortunately, I see many patients who fall into this category.

Trust me on this one. Every surgeon I know is anxious not to miss a structural problem. We as a surgical culture probably over-test our patients looking for a source of their pain. We not only don't want to miss something, we love to fix things. So if your surgeon is telling you that there is no structural problem, chances are that he or she is speaking the truth.

If there *is* a structural problem, decide to deal with it surgically or not. If it's a soft tissue problem or you have Mind Body Syndrome, it's important to accept that and move forward. If you can't let go of the idea that there must be a structural issue that's being missed, the ongoing anxiety regarding the source of your pain will hold you back.

CALMING THE CENTRAL NERVOUS SYSTEM

Regardless of whether your pain is from an identifiable source, the soft tissues, or a manifestation of MBS, your central nervous system must be "calmed down" before you can be treated. Here's why: physical therapy is usually part of the treatment for pain, no matter the source. It involves stretching and strengthening your muscles and ligaments, a process that requires significant force from your physical therapist in order to be effective. This manipulation of your inflamed tissues is painful at the very least; if the nervous system is also "fired up," it will be intolerable.

To start the process of calming your system, look at the DOCC program and consider how to apply it to your own situation. This chapter covers the first four parts of the program:

- Sleep
- Medications
- Education
- Goal Setting

All four of these factors affect the central nervous system, and they all need to be addressed. Leaving even one out will negatively affect your outcome. (Note: a fifth—stress management—is also a crucial part of decreasing the sensitivity of the nervous system. The whole middle part of this book will be devoted to that issue.)

Sleep

In treating chronic back pain, sleep is the trump card. All of the other variables affect sleep and sleep affects the other variables. I will see my patients back frequently specifically to check on sleep. If you have sleep issues, you should do the same with your own doctor. Not sleeping well is not an option in the successful treatment of chronic pain.

It's common to experience more pain at night than during the day since there are not as many distractions. There are multiple strategies to obtain a good night's sleep regardless of whether you are experiencing pain. They include:

- Sleep hygiene
- Medications
- Stress management at bedtime
- Treatment of an underlying sleep disorder

Sleep Hygiene

Sleep hygiene is a term that's used to describe a group of strategies that give you a better chance of getting a good night's sleep. In the context of chronic pain, these strategies usually need to be supplemented with medications, but they are nonetheless important.

First of all, you must be pro-active in getting a full eight hours of sleep. Allowing yourself to just lie in your bed not sleeping night after night is unacceptable. You may not see any results from your efforts initially, but your persistence will be rewarded in the end.

Many adults feel they can get by with much less sleep than what's recommended. The percent of adults who do not experience a consistent full night's sleep is estimated at around 35-40%. Some type of sleep disturbance is an issue for over 60 million Americans.[1]

In my surgeon's world it's somewhat of a perverse badge of honor to see how hard you can work with only five or six hours of sleep a night. This can and does become a way of life. However, at that point you no longer know what it's like to function regularly (i.e., with enough sleep). Your quality of life is compromised, but you are unaware of the extent to which this is the case. Some of the sleep hygiene concepts are:[2]

- Don't get into bed until you are ready to fall asleep. Watch TV, read, etc. in another room.
- Do not drink any caffeine after noon.
- Minimize alcohol intake in the evening—alcohol helps you to fall asleep but not stay asleep.
- Avoid heavy exercise in the evenings.
- Remove any clocks from the room.
- Do something relaxing just before going to bed.
- If you are hungry have a light snack.
- Concentrate on relaxing each muscle group in your body from head to toe.

The older you are, the more important it may become to practice good sleep hygiene. The ability to get a good night's sleep takes a definite downturn around age twenty-five and a larger downturn at age forty-five.

Sleep Medications

Nothing can really happen in the context of the DOCC structure until you are regularly getting enough sleep. (Exhaustion makes it impossible for anyone to concentrate long enough to engage in the program.) For those with chronic pain, this probably sounds impossible. You may think, how can I sleep with the intensity of the pain I am experiencing? It's a distinct problem and usually does require an aggressive medication approach.

If you're having sleep problems, work carefully with your doctor to figure out which sleep medication is best for you. Once you've started taking it, check with him or her every five to seven days —either at follow-up appointments or via phone— to report back on how things are going. If the first treatment plan isn't working, adjustments should be made promptly so that eventually you're sleeping well within three to four weeks. This is the kind of aggressive, solution-oriented approach that I've found is most effective.

If your doctor resists this kind of follow-up, do not back down. Calmly explain that getting sleep is a central part of your recovery program, one that you are taking seriously. Of course, if he/she still resists, don't be afraid to find another physician.

(Note: in dealing with sleep problems, some physicians opt for treating depression first, which does improve sleep. However, in my opinion this takes far too long.)

There are several categories of sleep medications and two basic strategies in terms of how they work. I am including them here to give you an idea of the wealth of options available. One group has a direct effect in that they will simply induce sleep. The other group includes medications that are intended for other problems but have drowsiness as a side effect. Sleep can be obtained by taking advantage of this side effect.

In addition to sleep medication, it can be helpful to take a slow-release narcotic, which will last for eight to twelve hours, to help with pain. I don't like narcotics specifically to get a patient to sleep, but they lessen the pain enough to allow the sleep medications to work. Narcotics are covered later in this chapter.

Here are the different types of sleep medications:

- Sedative-hypnotics
  - With anti-anxiety properties: Valium, Klonopin, Xanax, Halcion, Ativan, etc.
  - Without anti-anxiety properties: Ambien, Lunesta, Sonata
- Antidepressants with drowsiness as a side effect
  - Tricyclics: Amitryptiline (Elavil), Nortriptyline (Pamelor)
  - Non-SSRI: Remeron, Trazodone
- Anti-psychotics with drowsiness as a side effect
  - Seroquel, Risperdol
- Melatonin agonists
  - Melatonin, Rozeram
- Antihistamines
  - Benadryl
  - Over-the-counter sleep aids

I won't go into the pros and cons of each medication—that is something to discuss with your doctor. But know that one of the above will work for you if used correctly. Pain is not a reason to lose a night's sleep.

Stress Management at Bedtime

When you are under stress your brain is on a Formula One racetrack. It may feel hard to slow down your racing thoughts during the day, and next to impossible at night in the quiet of your bedroom. A good part of this book is focused on stress management. As you more effectively process your stress, your sleep will definitely improve. However, as lack of sleep in and of itself is a major stress, this is a little tricky. Again, just getting to sleep with meds is the starting point. As a next step, I suggest doing the writing exercises outlined in Chapters 7 and 9 at bedtime. Many sleep specialists are encouraging these types of cognitive behavioral exercises at bedtime as a sleep strategy. Keep a writing pad next to your bed so you can write if you wake up in the middle of the night—this will help you quickly fall back asleep. It's remarkable how effective writing is in slowing down whirlpools of obsessive thoughts.

Diagnosing Sleep Disorders

It has been said that only five percent of patients with sleep issues ever receive an adequate evaluation of their issues by a physician.[3] This is unfortunate, because lack of sleep is such a common problem. The term commonly applied to trouble getting a good night's sleep is insomnia, but there are over one hundred additional sleep disorders in existence. Two major disorders are restless leg syndrome and sleep apnea.

If sleep medication, pain medication, and stress management do not help your sleep over a reasonable period of time, then you might want to get further testing by a sleep specialist to establish a firm diagnosis.

Medication Management

When you're experiencing chronic back pain, your day-to-day routine is often completely upended. It may be difficult to even get out of bed and move around the house, never mind going to work. The first goal of the DOCC program is to improve your ability to function, which in itself is usually followed by some degree of pain relief. Taking medication, often on a short-term basis, helps you to become more functional so that you can fully engage in your care. Here we will discuss some of the common types of meds taken by those experiencing chronic pain: for pain, anxiety, depression, and muscle spasms.

As with sleep medication, work with your doctor to find the right pain medication for you. Speak in a direct way with him/her to find out the goal of each medication and its potential side effects. Your physician may prescribe multiple meds over time, but this is generally a bad idea—taking a number of them at the same time increases your risk of experiencing side effects and having a worse quality of life. It's not uncommon for meds to be prescribed to treat the side effect of another medication, and on and on. So it's important to take responsibility for minimizing them. Physicians are often too busy and may not take the time to sort out the implications of multiple side effects and/or possible adverse drug interactions.

I've included a general overview of the different types of meds here so you can have an informed conversation with your doctor about the alternatives.

Decreasing Pain: Narcotics

While I am not a great fan of taking narcotics on an ongoing basis, there is one situation where I think they may be useful within the DOCC structure: when patients can't function at the most basic activity level. In this case, taking narcotics for adequate pain control can help significantly. Though it does not solve the chronic pain problem, this allows patients to move around more easily in the short term and start the recovery process.

Narcotics all have similar effects and side effects, they just vary in how they are administered and how long they last. In other words, codeine and heroin have the same effects and side effects, but heroin is much more concentrated and is generally taken intravenously. Codeine is much less concentrated and is taken by mouth.

There are two basic categories of narcotics: they are either direct derivatives of opium or artificially synthesized. Examples of direct opium derivatives are:

- Morphine
- Heroin
- Codeine

Examples of semi-synthetics are:

- Oxycodone (Percocet, Percodan, Tylox)
- Hyrocodone (Vicodin, Loracet, Norco)
- Dilaudid
- Tramadol (Ultram)
- Darvocet
- Methadone
- Fentanyl
- Demerol

Note that it's important to distinguish whether a narcotic is long acting. (Some in this category are encased in a slow-release outer coating.) A common one is Oxycontin, which is just short-acting oxycodone in a time-release capsule. It's critical not to chew a time-release narcotic because if you do so the amount of drug ingested over a short time can be lethal. Other narcotics are long acting just by the nature of the chemistry of the drug. The classic example is methadone, which has an extended duration. In fact, it lasts so long that if taken too often it can quickly build up and also become lethal.

The Downside of Narcotics

I am careful about long-term narcotics, but not for moral reasons—I spent about five years actively prescribing them. Rather, I'm cautious because there's a significant downside to these medications. For one, there's the tolerance factor: the liver becomes more efficient in breaking down the drug and it takes more of the drug to have the same effect. Secondly, many patients just don't feel that great on narcotics. They complain of fuzzy thinking, which they sometimes haven't even realized until they come off them. Thirdly, narcotics *are* addictive. It's a true addiction, and therefore extremely difficult to break.

The most disturbing aspect of narcotics of all is that they affect the sensitivity of the nervous system. The term for this process is "up-sensitization" or "opioid-induced hyperalgesia." In rat studies, it's been shown that repeated administration of narcotics causes them to be more sensitive to pain stimuli.[4] It's unclear exactly why this happens. It may stem from the fact that narcotics cause changes in the glial cells in the brain and spinal cord, which insulate the nerve sheaths.

At the start of the DOCC program, I never stop or decrease a patient's current narcotic intake. Instead, we first deal with sleep and then stress—when you're in chronic pain, your life is difficult enough without the additional strain of coming off pain meds. Once you develop decent stress management skills, *then* you can start a gradual tapering off of the meds. The tapering off rarely occurs before six months of being engaged in the program, and usually it takes twelve to eighteen months for a given patient to be really ready to stop taking them altogether. This should be a clear goal in your mind.

Decreasing Pain: Non-Narcotics

Anti-inflammatory medications such as ibuprofen decrease pain in two different ways. The direct relief of pain occurs any time you take the drug. A decrease in inflammation requires a sustained dose over a number of weeks.

Direct pain relief from anti-inflammatories works well and is predictable. All of us have taken them for a headache, sore back, etc. Studies have consistently shown that they work as well as lower potency narcotics such as Tylenol with codeine and Vicodin. What's more, a recent study of 336 children with arm fractures showed that the failure rate for pain control was 30% with codeine and only 20% with ibuprofen. In addition, the patients had more undesirable side effects with the codeine. Both parents and their children were more satisfied with the ibuprofen.[5]

Decreasing inflammation is a much different process than direct pain relief. An anti-inflammatory needs to be taken for at least two or three weeks for its full effect to kick in. Often patients find it difficult to sustain a pharmacological dose for the required

43

period, and skip a day or two. But even missing a day will markedly diminish the drug's effectiveness.

Examples of anti-inflammatories include:

- Ibuprofen (Advil)
- Naprosyn (Aleve)
- Indocin
- Relafen

Tylenol, which is not an anti-inflammatory, is also an effective pain reliever. The drawback is that it has the predictable effect of causing kidney and/or liver failure if you take too much. It's recommended not to take more than four grams per day. And be careful—there are so many medications that have Tylenol as an ingredient that it's easy to inadvertently exceed this dose.

Decreasing Anxiety

Anxiolytics (Valium-type medications) work very well for decreasing anxiety. That's the good news and the bad news. They do provide quick and significant relief of severe anxiety. It's impossible to reduce anxiety if you are consumed by it, so short-term relief from anxiolytics can be very helpful to get you started. The bad news is that they are very addicting and hard to discontinue. The addiction is not a true addiction; it's more of a dependency. In other words, you become dependent on the meds to allay your anxiety, which will quickly flare up as you come off of them. Therefore meds are not the definitive answer and should only be used in conjunction with an aggressive program to treat anxiety.

Nervous system medicines like Neurontin and Lyrica work directly on the nervous system by decreasing the excitability of the nerves. One side effect of these drugs is that as they calm down the nervous system they may help lessen anxiety and so may also have a positive effect on sleep. The main reason they were designed was to treat seizures, but they are also used to treat nerve pain. It's unpredictable who might obtain relief of the nerve pain, but when it occurs it can be dramatic.

Antidepressant medications are very effective in treating chronic pain-associated depression in the short term. Many patients are so depressed and beaten up by their pain that they cannot move forward without meds. While antidepressants are helpful for depression, though, they aren't a substitute for the work on stress management we will cover in this book.

Also, it should be made clear to you whether the medication you are taking for depression is meant to induce sleep or primarily meant to treat your depression and thereby indirectly improve your sleep. Some of these medications induce drowsiness; others will stimulate you.

Anti–muscle spasm medications create controversy in my mind in the context of treating chronic pain; I have never seen them be very useful. Although the side effects are not severe, they just don't seem to have much effect other than making you a little drowsy. I am not adamantly against them, I just think they make things a little more complicated. Note that Soma is a drug to be avoided. It metabolizes into a short-acting barbiturate and is extremely habit-forming.

Education

Educating yourself about your care is a critical part of the DOCC program. If you're having anxiety, you can decrease it by learning about what's involved in taking charge of your own care. There's a lot of detailed information and the education process requires a strong commitment, but think of it as your responsibility in the recovery process. Start with your specific condition, and then find out about the different treatments available, both operative and non-operative. Reading this book is an important step, and there are many other resources.

It has been pointed out to me for years that patients will often make decisions about major spine surgery with less research than they do when buying a new car. I think this might be because patients do tend to trust their doctors to make the right decision for them. However, physicians are not able to really understand your life and pain in a busy office setting. Not even your own family can completely understand what's going on in your head. Surgeons also are not trained in all the variables involved in the evolution of chronic pain. Take charge of your decisions. Do not turn them over to anyone.

Goal Setting

As we live our lives, whether we have chronic pain or not, it's easy to fall into a "surviving and fixing" mind-set. You go along and deal with any problems in a reactive way. When was the last time you thought about living your life based on a vision instead of just getting by?

Running your life should be like running a business. While this may seem impossible in the context of chronic pain, there's no time when it's more vital. There are multiple components in your life that have to come together in order for it to be successful. Although the variables are different from business, the principles are the same. You must first have an idea of where you are, where you want to go, and how you are going to accomplish what you need to. Then you have to develop the tools necessary to get there. Two of the basic tools are being organized and having good communication skills.

This section provides exercises to get you started with identifying your goals. More detailed goal-setting exercises are presented in Chapter 9, Stage IV.

The Three Questions

To start the goal-setting process, first write down the three questions: Where am I now? Where do I want to go? How am I going to get there?

Figuring out where you are (first answer) is critical. To answer this question in terms of a business, you would start by assessing your current skills and assets. In the context of chronic pain, this step entails gaining an understanding of your problem and what you can do about it. It's the only way to move forward.

The second answer, where you want to go, has to be specific. The answers, "I just want to get rid of my pain" or "I just want my life back" are not helpful—they lack any type of direction or purpose. It's critical to think about your answer carefully and either regain your previous direction in life or establish a new one based on your current situation. If you continue without a compass, you are giving your life over to your pain.

For number three, how are you going to get there, you need a plan. First, consider a business that had no direction or plan. There would be no focus of energy and lots of anxiety and frustration. It's the same for you. Removing those distractions (anxiety and frustration) can have a significant calming effect. So not only is your nervous system calmer, you are able to pursue the treatments that will calm it down even more.

In answering the three questions, keep in mind that it's common in our culture to feel that if you had more of "X," then you would be happier. "X" can include more money, better-behaved children, a nicer boss, etc. It can also include "less pain." I don't disagree that good circumstances are better than bad circumstances. However, many if not most circumstances are beyond our control. In Eastern cultures, it's often the other way around. If you can first attain a peace of mind regardless of your circumstances, then you will have the energy to create the life that you want. Part of this is coming up with a vision that doesn't require outside changes and steadily working toward attaining it.

It borders on insanity to think that each one of many things would line up well enough for you to be perfectly happy. Blame it on our culture, which drives us hard to achieve this utopia. But your peace of mind cannot be dependent on your external circumstances. Trying to control everything is a waste of the emotional energy you need to create the life you desire. Physicians have a tendency to get into this type of endless delayed-gratification mode with some vague feeling that if enough of our circumstances were perfect, we'd be happier. Every day brings on a new set of pretty intense stressors, though. That's why I've written down a phrase to myself, "Don't let anyone or anything, anywhere, anytime, or anyplace take away my ability to enjoy my day."

Anger and Making Plans

We covered the role that anger plays in chronic pain in Chapter 1, and will discuss how to get rid of it in later chapters. In the context of goal setting and organizing your life, it's important to be aware of how anger can hold you back.

If you are angry, in a reactive mode, it's difficult to develop a plan. A good metaphor for your anger is how they handle elephants in India. When the elephants are very small, they train them to stay in one place by tying one foot to a stake. When the elephant has turned into a huge adult, it will still be held in place by the same type of small stake. The animals have been programmed to think of the stake as something that cannot be pulled up. Anger is similar. It anchors you down in one place and you cannot move forward until you understand that this restraint exists. Then you can break free. Make this part of your plan.

Social Isolation

Goal setting is a critical part of your becoming pain-free for several reasons. One is that it's common, if not the rule, for patients suffering from chronic pain to become socially isolated. As you become more isolated, a higher percentage of your consciousness is spent experiencing the pain, feeling the frustrations associated with trying to find a cause, and trying to escape it. These anxiety/pain/frustration circuits turn monstrous, taking over your formerly productive life. I routinely ask patients about their social life and they *always* just shake their heads with a sad look. If you're in the same situation, know that you cannot will your way out of this. You need to create achievable goals to break out of this particular prison.

A study done in 2003 showed that when study volunteers were met with perceived social isolation, the same part of the brain lit up on a functional MRI as it did when they experienced physical pain.[6] The same result occurred with every participant every time. This shows yet another "loop" that happens with chronic pain: you become isolated and experience even more pain than before. Then the increased pain makes it less likely that you'll reach out to your friends and family. In fact, not only do patients *not* reach out, they often lash out at those they need for support, driving them away. We all need each other—don't let chronic pain take that away from you.

Implementing Your Goals: Get Organized

To stay on top of your goals and your treatment plan, it's important to be organized about it. This involves checking everything on a weekly basis and updating as needed. You may think that you're not an organized person and there's nothing to be done about that. But that's not true: organization is a learned skill.

Organizational skills have never come easily to me. In fact, I have ADHD. I have been legendary since high school for losing things. Because of the inherently tight structure of medical school and residency, I functioned very well there. A good work ethic has also been helpful. But I when I entered private practice, organizing my time and efforts instantly became much more difficult.

When I went into private practice in 1986, I realized within a couple of weeks that there was no longer a tight structure guiding me. There were so many things coming at me from so many different directions. Part of my identity had always been, "I am just not an organized person," but that needed to change, and fast.

I happened to pick up a book, *The Organized Executive* by Stephanie Winston, and was quickly able to put the principles she presented into practice.[7] Although the book did not solve all of my problems, I became very organized. My first focus was and still is to make sure that I follow up on every test I order on my patients. Over time I was able to keep up on almost everything I needed to do to provide good follow-up care; very few things fell through the cracks. There's no way I would've figured this out without help.

Later, my brother encouraged me to look at an organizational system created by David Allen, author of the book, *Getting Things Done*.[8] Being that he was my little brother, I didn't jump at his suggestion initially. However, I noted that by using Allen's precepts, he'd gone from middle manager at his company to vice-president within three years. He's now a senior vice-president. I finally read the book and went to a seminar given by the author a month later.

I was blown away—Allen's concepts are brilliant. His core strategy is to define any task that takes more than two minutes as a project. Everything in your life is filed away in a simple enough system that it is easily retrievable. The analogy he uses is putting all of our "to do" lists on the "hard drive." Most of us keep our tasks in the RAM (random access memory), which means it keeps spinning around in our heads. This not only doesn't work, it wears us out.

Becoming organized allows you to engage in as many projects as needed to accomplish your goals. In this way it's possible to change the way you think about how you approach your whole life. Consider that it's common for us to be "sequential thinkers." We think, "When I feel better, I'll do this," or "When I'm under less stress, I'll have the willpower to exercise," or "When I retire, I'll really enjoy my life." You can get stuck in a cycle of putting things off and inadvertently become a victim of your own circumstances.

If you outline and organize all your projects, however, it's possible to *stop* thinking sequentially. Instead of waiting to accomplish what you want, you just have to figure out "the one next step." That is a David Allen term which in and of itself has changed my life. He describes a weekly "mind sweep," when you review what's on the "hard drive" and pull it out on your "to do" list. Using Allen's book, I have been able to accomplish things I never would have thought possible for me. For example, this book would not have been written without my understanding of his organizational strategies.

Getting organized in the context of your chronic pain problem accomplishes several things. 1) It enables you to decrease your stress by gaining better control of your environment. 2) It clears creative space in your head so you can better solve any problems. 3) Finally, it helps you to move forward on as many fronts as necessary, whereas keeping your "to do" list in your head actually reinforces any patterns of obsessive thinking you may be prone to.

There are many organizational systems. If organization is not your strong suit, do a little research and find one that is right for you.

GAINING PERSPECTIVE

At the close of this chapter, I'd like to address the importance of retaining perspective on life. In planning and living your life, nothing is more crucial than perspective. In my own, I've found a concept that is immensely helpful in this regard. It's a project called "The Journey of the 1,000 Moons," created by my friend, the artist Ernesto Sanchez. The "1,000 Moons" helps me maintain my equilibrium in the midst of the chaos inherent in being a complex spinal deformity surgeon. The concept can be used to bring balance to any chaotic life, including one that's touched by chronic pain. I have two of his moon sculptures hanging in my office.

Here is Ernesto's description of the project:

If you count the moon cycles you will experience in your lifetime, by the time you reach 77 years of age you will have experienced one thousand. As we live these years, how often do we stop and think about the presence of the moon in our lives and on the earth?

51

To honor the inspirational force that the moon has on my life, I began an art project called "The Journey of 1,000 Moons." The goal is simple: to make 1,000 moons. The moons are cast in gypsum and hand painted. Like our lives, each moon is unique. For every journey there is a path, and on the path are points of inspiration, illumination, and revelation. But you cannot experience these unless you take the journey.

The Journey of 1,000 Moons reminds us that while the energetic dance between the moon and the earth has endured for billions of years, each of our individual lives is but a brief flash of illumination—only 1,000 moons.

Ernesto's ritual "moon burning" ceremony—in which he burns one of his moon sculptures—can represent many things to the participant. For my patients there's the obvious metaphor of watching your life go up in flames living in chronic pain, or it can also symbolize letting go of your past and moving forward.

Ernesto has been an inspiration to me with his commitment to the arts as a way of elevating the spirit. I hope the "1,000 Moons" is helpful in your journey back to a full, rich, and pain-free life.

SUMMARY AND NEXT STEPS

At this point, you should have a handle on your anatomic issues. Also, one of the following has occurred: 1) you've been told that nothing can be done surgically or the potential benefit of surgery is not worth the risk, or 2) you've undergone surgery. If it's choice 2, the surgery may have not lived up to your expectations.

Remember that your path out of pain involves the following variables and ALL of them must be addressed for a successful outcome:

- Education
- Sleep
- Stress

- Medications
- Goal Setting
- Physical Rehabilitation

We have now covered much of the DOCC program. You have learned about the various factors that affect pain, including: 1) Your pain will not decrease until you are regularly experiencing a restful night's sleep. 2) Medications are critical in the early stages for improving sleep, decreasing pain, and addressing anxiety; as you progress on your journey, medications eventually will not be necessary. 3) Although goal setting plays a more prominent role later in the healing process than at the outset, it's helpful to start considering it early on.

Learning how to deal with the stress caused by living in chronic pain is at the heart of the DOCC program. The rest of this book will address the various ways that pain has torn apart your life and offer additional concrete tools for coping with it. Once your nervous system has calmed down somewhat, then rehabilitation and physical conditioning become the final focus of the process. Rehab and fitness are described in detail in Chapter 10.

CHAPTER 3

Stress Management

At this point in the book we've established that stress plays a major role in chronic pain. Pain itself is a major stressor, as is the inability to recover. The resultant anxiety and frustration are intense. Add in the normal stresses of everyday life—work, relationships, travel—and your stress levels can go into the stratosphere. Stress hormones, including adrenaline and cortisol, become elevated. These chemicals cause your heart to race and your senses to be on constant alert. Your nervous system gets fired up and your pain increases. The entire process wears you down.

The main goal of this chapter is to organize your thinking about stress management. Think in terms of your energy level. There are two variables: 1) building up your energy reserves, and 2) plugging the drain. The second step is the most critical.

It's important to engage in activities that build up your energy reserves. This is the positive aspect of managing stress. Examples are adequate sleep; consistent exercise; hobbies; enjoyable time with friends and family; setting boundaries; positive conflict resolution; and time alone. These nurturing activities are the focus of most stress management literature and seminars. However, they cannot be done in isolation. The other aspect of managing stress revolves around minimizing the effects of negative emotions, which are caused by—for the most part—anxiety fueled by anger. What's often missed in the understanding of stress management is that the two major parts—building up energy and avoiding the energy drain of anxiety—are *not* linked. In other words, you can gain more energy and yet still suffer from anxiety.

A third aspect of managing stress is what I call "the myth of self-esteem." We are programmed in our society to believe that if we have enough of the good things in life we will gain more self-worth, be "happy," and, by definition, have less anxiety. We work very hard on gaining achievements, possessions, and experiences, and we think they'll propel us to an elevated state of existence. But unfortunately, by pursuing self-esteem to find happiness, you are using a rational way to deal with completely irrational, unresponsive neurological circuits. Not only is it ineffective, it's exhausting, and throughout the entire process, circuits of anxiety driven by anger will suck the life right out of you.

The real goal in our pursuit of genuine happiness is to feel less anxious. Anxiety is the deepest survival emotion. It's intended to make us feel vulnerable and helpless, which of course we hate. We cannot survive without anxiety yet we aren't taught the basic skills needed to process it.

So picture your life as a bathtub. The water flowing through the faucet represents the enjoyable, rejuvenating parts of your life that create energy. Then picture an unusually large drain that represents anxiety and anger. If the drain is wide open, it won't matter how much water you put into the tub, it will never fill up. It will be impossible to build up your energy reserves to a level where you can enjoy your life. If you never deal with your anxiety and anger, the psychic drain will be continual.

Or, picture yourself trying to cross a large body of water in a slowly sinking boat. You can't navigate the boat and bail at the same time. Even if it were possible, it certainly detracts from the enjoyment of the trip. Your only focus is on survival instead of having a good time. You're exhausted.

Now see yourself running the bath water with the drain closed. You've learned how to address your anxiety—and anger-related stress—so you can relax into the tub and calm your senses. Likewise, the boat is no longer sinking, so you can sit back and enjoy the experience. You have energy not only to survive but also to live life fully.

It's critical to plug the metaphorical drain in your life. Once it's plugged, then not only will the tub fill, it will overflow to others around you. You will see over the next few chapters that the "drain-plugging" methods are simple and effective; we all should have been taught them from elementary school.

I personally was able to implement effective stress management tactics at around age fifty. It took a long time, but I finally got there. Now I would conservatively estimate that I have two to three times the amount of energy I had when I was in high school. It's also not the hyper, wired energy I felt back then, which was very dependent on external factors. Now it comes from a much deeper and more stable place within me.

Learning how to better cope with stress has a dramatic effect on your quality of life: it improves your relationships, helps you make better decisions, and, most critically for chronic pain patients, calms your nervous system. The calmer your nervous system, the greater chances that your pain will decrease.

REACTIONS TO STRESS

One of the most important principles I've learned about stress is that it's not the source of our problems in life. Rather, it's our reaction to stress that causes unpleasant emotions and drains our energy.

A stressor is any situation that causes a reaction. Although in this chapter I refer to difficult situations, keep in mind that positive events such as weddings, buying a new house, new career changes, etc. are also stressors.

In any scenario, your reaction to (i.e., your thoughts about) a stressor is the most important part of the picture. Why? Because people often identify with their thoughts. It's been pointed out for many centuries, however, that you are not your thoughts. When you encounter a stressor, try seeing your thoughts in reaction to the stressor as separate from who you are.

Let's take an example of your child coming home late again well after his curfew. As you confront him, he might "talk back," letting you know in a very efficient manner just what kind of human being you are. Predictably, and understandably, you react with anger.

In this situation, the stressor was your child coming in late and then responding to your confrontation in an aggressive, defensive way. The situation in and of itself is not an energy drain. After all, you weren't physically harmed. Rather, it's your reaction of anger that drains your energy and brings you down. If you don't separate your reaction from the stressor, it all ends up feeling like one ugly event. Then as most people do, you identify with your thoughts. So now you are "the angry parent." By developing an awareness of the various parts of the interaction, you can more effectively deal with it.

As you are the adult, a better response would have been to not engage in a conversation while you were upset. Later in the chapter, we'll talk about how when a situation or person makes you angry, it's because a patterned response was set off within you. It's not the circumstance or other person causing the angry response, it's your own thoughts. Once you have defused your response (by waiting a few hours/overnight) you can then talk the situation over in a civil manner. Teenagers are not reliable and they tend to lie when pressed. Remember when you were a teenager? Have you ever noticed that an issue *never* gets solved when one or both parties are upset? Handling a situation poorly has fallout that can carry over into other aspects of your relationship for days, weeks, months, or even years. Instead of putting your relationship at risk, take a step back before exploding.

As important as it is to wait before reacting, I know it's not easy. Implementing this concept is still my greatest personal challenge.

Another example I frequently use in clinic is driving. I ask patients, "If you're cut off in traffic by another car, and then the other driver flips you off, what would cause you to feel stressed and possibly get angry? You weren't involved in an accident. Would it be the situation or your reaction to it that upset you?"

If you drive, there's no way to avoid interacting with bad drivers. You can't control that. Why would you give someone who you feel is inconsiderate the power to ruin your day?

An important step in dealing with stressful situations is to create an *awareness* of the components of the circumstances. You can do this by: 1) separating your reaction (thoughts) from a given stressor, and 2) separating yourself from your thoughts. The end result is that you and the stressor are on "opposite sides of the room" and the reaction (your thoughts) to the stressor is in the "middle of the room." By making these separations, you can clearly see your reaction to the stressor as a separate entity and handle the situation in a more productive way. You're giving yourself a choice.

Anxiety and anger are not who you are. They are thoughts and resultant emotions that exist in you *separate* from your value system and how you choose to live your life. Until you can separate these emotions from your core identity, the drain in the tub will be wide open. The goal of this chapter is to help you create a personal awareness of your psychic drain. You will then learn tools that effectively put a permanent plug in it.

The Stress of Pain—"The Terrifying Triad"

There's a good chance that if you're reading this book right now, your life is not exactly as you'd like it to be. You're experiencing pain that is significantly altering your quality of life and you aren't happy about it. The medical profession hasn't provided an adequate explanation of why you're in pain; you've been offered multiple treatments that initially raised your hopes of a better life, yet the treatments didn't result in any lasting relief. As the pain drags on and your expectations aren't met, you become more and more anxious and frustrated. In addition, your nervous system is being pounded by pain impulses. It's an intersection of the neurological pathways of pain, anxiety, and anger. This is what I refer to as "the terrifying triad."

One way that anxiety occurs is when a basic human need such as air, food, or water isn't met. This causes us to take action to meet the need and allay our anxiety. If we can't take action, anxiety escalates to fear and ultimately anger. A good analogy is if you were forced to hold your hand over the hot burner of a stove. Being in chronic pain is like being unable to remove your hand from the burner. In this situation, you'd experience the sequence of anxiety, fear, anger, and, after enough time, rage that one of your basic human needs—not being in pain—isn't being met.

Of course, there are other sources of stress besides pain. Pain sets off anxiety and anger but now other life stresses such as having a difficult boss, tumultuous relationships, difficulty with finances, etc. become connected to the pain pathways. When you're under a lot of stress and experience more pain, it's *not* imaginary or "psychological." The stress and pain pathways in your body have now been linked together, so the pain is real. It's been demonstrated on functional MRIs that when you're under chronic stress, the corresponding pain areas in your brain become abnormally activated. More distress neurons fire per stimulus than when you are calm. Your brain is "on fire."[1]

As I work with patients on the DOCC project for a while, they become aware of the link between stress and pain. They see that when their stress reaches a certain point, there's a corresponding increase in their pain. The pain can be so severe that I frequently feel compelled to reorder diagnostic tests, but they rarely reveal anything of significance.

Stress can be reduced when I'm able to surgically remove the source of pain (for a structural injury), but if a patient has been in chronic pain before the surgery, there tends to be a permanent increase in the patient's level of anxiety and frustration. Even when the structural problem is solved, there are so many other ways for these pathways to remain stimulated. There's the stress of finding a new job with a history of a back problem; a family that's suffered the impact of your frustrations; and the challenge of getting back into shape physically. That's why it's so important for patients to address anxiety and anger before *and* after their procedure. Letting your anxiety/anger circuits run wild can be ruinous; conversely, the rewards of breaking up these pathways are great.

Stress Management—Basic Concepts

There are many misconceptions about stress management. In my experience, most of us don't have a clear idea of how to manage our stress. My tool from early high school was to always "think positive" and just be tough. No one could hurt me. I wouldn't allow myself to get angry, no matter what the circumstances. I didn't even know what anxiety was; I did not become a major spinal deformity surgeon by being anxious. I could endure and charge through almost any adversity.

I recall that a few people I dated in college used to refer to me as "the brick." I could put a wall around anything. I knew at the time that from their perspective, it was not complimentary. However, I took it as somewhat of a perverse compliment.

During every summer and breaks throughout medical school I worked in the construction field. I spent most of the time framing, pouring and finishing concrete slabs, and doing some finish carpentry. One summer afternoon I was framing on a hot day in Napa Valley. I hadn't had much sleep the night before. It was one of my personal challenges to consistently sink a 16-penny nail with two swings of the hammer and occasionally one. At one point, I was bending over and holding a stud against the floor plate when I took a full swing with my 28-ounce framing hammer. On the way down the hammer glanced off an upright piece of plastic plumbing and landed squarely on my left thumb. The pain was so intense that I almost passed out. I stood up, looked at my mangled thumb, wrapped it up in a rag, and went back to work without a word. My boss, who'd been standing just ten feet away, thought I was out of my mind. In retrospect I probably was. I was really tough.

I later learned that being tough, however, doesn't yield a full and satisfying life. Neither does positive thinking. Toughness is actually a variant of positive thinking, and there are prices to pay for both. Being tough and/or positive all the time is like pushing a rock up an endless hill. Eventually you just get worn out.

My toughness and positive thinking eventually caught up with me. In 1988, I started going into a long period of burnout and depression. Later I began to have severe anxiety reactions that progressed into full-blown panic attacks. By 1997, I had developed an obsessive-compulsive disorder, and within a few years I was seriously suicidal. I didn't survive the ordeal because I had any ray of hope; my darkness was complete. Instead, it was family ties that pulled me through. I had two physician friends whose lives were severely impacted when their fathers committed suicide during their teenage years. I simply made a decision not to abandon my son. By 2003 I had pulled out of my dark place in a dramatic way. I did it by using the tools that I am presenting in this book. Now I feel like I've been given a second chance at a life, one that I couldn't visualize during those difficult years.

Everything I'm sharing with you I've learned through an extremely harsh experience. Much of it could've been avoided if I hadn't made some significant mistakes along the way. I feel strongly that if I'd been taught stress management principles in school, my life would have been dramatically different. Here are some of those principles:

- Managing stress is a learned skill.
- Anxiety is an emotion that never gets better with time. Untreated, it always gets worse.
- No human being escapes this relentless progression of anxiety—no one!! Some are just better at disguising it for a while.

- From what I've seen, the number one factor that determines success in life is the ability to process adversity and be resilient (which is much different than being "tough").
- What most of us learn from elementary through high school are only survival skills—and they are not skills. How many of us were ever taught basic stress management principles? Unless these principles are learned and implemented we will continue to reinforce dysfunctional coping methods.
- We are programmed by our families' coping patterns, which are typically not very effective.
- Anger = loss of control. The need for control is caused by anxiety. Therefore the driving force behind anger is anxiety.
- Anger is at the core of obsessive behavior. Once my patients in pain become truly (and appropriately) angry, the whole nature of their interaction with their families and the medical system changes in a terrible way. They become focused on the pain and it runs their lives.
- Living a full life requires having a vision. As life beats us down, most of us lose that vision and gradually go into survival mode. Chronic pain greatly magnifies the problem. Getting that vision back in spite of the pain is critical.
- The centerpiece of dealing with stress is awareness. Awareness is the opposite of positive thinking. Positive thinking breeds thought suppression, while awareness connects us to our thoughts and to the details of our environment.

Pain is one of life's most difficult stressors. It's paradoxical that a beautifully designed system intended to protect you can also cause so much grief. The crushing aspect of chronic pain is that there appears to be no escape nor an end in sight.

The feeling of being trapped was familiar to Victor Frankel, a famous Jewish psychiatrist who survived WWII concentration camps. He wrote the classic book, *Man's Search for Meaning*.[2] It is striking that in spite of the extreme physical hardships Frankel endured, for him the most difficult part of the ordeal was not knowing if and when it was going to end—which is similar if not identical to what patients in chronic pain experience.

PROGRAMMING

I am a strong supporter of psychology, psychiatry, and any mental health professional who can provide insight into how to live a full and productive life. However, I want you to think differently about mental health for a moment. Consider it not in terms of talk therapy but in terms of "neurological programming." If you look carefully at your life, you'll see that many of your attitudes and behaviors are a direct result of adopting or rebelling against your family's patterns. We have all been "programmed" by our families, but it's possible to "reprogram" ourselves.

One day I happened to hit a nerve with a patient regarding his family patterns. Jim needed a back operation for a pinched nerve that was causing right leg pain. Moody and uncooperative, he hadn't followed up on anything we'd discussed in his appointments. I couldn't get him to engage with any of the stress management tools.

Finally I gave up. "Look," I said. "I'm going to cancel your surgery. I can't engage with you if you don't want to participate in learning the tools I'm trying to give you to get better. It's just the way I work." I had a sense that Jim's resistance to stress management stemmed from his background, so I also added, "We're all programmed by our past. For example, if you were raised in family that was active in the Ku Klux Klan, what do you think your belief system would be?" His fiancée suddenly burst out laughing hysterically. It didn't seem that funny to me, particularly since I was frustrated with his unwillingness to engage.

I thought I'd picked a completely random example. But Jim looked me in the eye and said, "My father and grandfather were Grand Knights in the Klan."

I did cancel the surgery. My theoretical example of family programming apparently hit home and Jim finally began to engage in the DOCC program. In the end, the surgery was rescheduled three months later and was successful in relieving his leg pain. He has made a great deal of progress with stress management skills because he shifted his thinking and came at the process from a difficult place. Jim's struggle to learn a better way to deal with stress borders on heroic. I hear from him every few months and he continues to evolve. His skills have created a better life for him, his wife, and their three small children. It *is* a high stakes game.

Once the reprogramming foundation is established, my patients work hard to apply its principles to their lives. The only patients I've seen that did not experience significant benefit from reprogramming exercises are the ones who did not fully engage on a long-term basis. With full engagement, success in eliminating your pain is probable, not just possible.

In the next three chapters we'll focus on anxiety, anger, and how the two feed off of and drive each other. We'll also explore potential solutions to the problem of the anxiety/anger axis.

My life has greatly benefited from learning how to deal with anxiety and anger. Ten years ago, my psychiatrist told me there was a way to live my life that I couldn't comprehend because I had never experienced it. It's difficult to learn something when you have no idea what it might be. I was able to open the door in 2003 and walk through it in 2006. I learned that it's not about being happy or depressed. It's not about constantly trying to "fix" myself. It's about plugging the drain of anxiety and anger and having the energy to create my life on my own terms. It's living with awareness and letting go. It's a much more interesting life.

CHAPTER 4
Anxiety

The ability to deal with anxiety in a healthy way is critical to anyone's quality of life, and it's even more important for someone in chronic pain. Patients in chronic pain typically have anxiety-related thoughts such as "What is the source of my pain?" "Why can't anyone figure out the problem?" "Will there be an end to this misery?" They also wonder if they will be able to support their families and/or whether they'll become drug addicted if they take pain medication. When no answers to these questions emerge, anxiety can escalate dramatically. With the nervous system "fired up," the pain worsens and the capacity to cope diminishes.

As human beings we are, by definition, anxious creatures. Anxiety levels vary from person to person (as does the ability to cover it up) but in general we all experience a good deal of anxiety. Think how much energy we expend on showing the world that we're not anxious. We want to look good to everyone and we also want to look good to ourselves.

Every human being has anxiety "hard-wired" into his or her brain. It keeps us out of trouble by signaling "danger ahead." As such, it's a necessary emotion for survival. Anxiety represents the feelings of vulnerability and helplessness which we are programmed to avoid at almost any cost. And while we have a deep instinct to avoid anxiety itself, as well as the danger it may signal, we are confronted with it on a daily basis.

The more anxiety we experience, the more it produces neurologic pathways that become "etched" into our brains. Typically, we're not taught effective ways to stop the progression of these circuits, so we end up using dysfunctional coping patterns that detract from our quality of life. It's my personal feeling that most mental health issues have their basis in progressive anxiety. From my perspective, progressive anxiety looks like a "programming" problem, not a psychological issue.

THE CREATION OF ANXIETY

To further understand anxiety and learn how to handle it effectively, it helps to break it down into parts.

To experience anxiety, you must first have an anxiety-producing thought. For example, if you stepped off of a curb and almost got hit by a car, your heart might race and your stomach might clench even though nothing touched you. It was the thought that you might get hit that caused the secretion of chemicals, eliciting the physical response. I think of the sequence as a "psychological reflex," one that sparks a constellation of feelings in addition to anxiety such as fear, frustration, or anger.

In another example, picture yourself lying on a sunny beach in Hawaii thinking about how glad you are to be on vacation. You feel relaxed because the happy thoughts lead your body to secrete chemicals similar to the drug Valium. Different thoughts can radically change your emotions and physical condition. If you're on the same beach thinking about how poorly your boss has been treating you, how are you going to feel? Probably frustrated and a bit angry. Even though you're on a gorgeous beach you can't relax. Again, it's the thought, not the circumstances you're in, that determines your emotional state. If you continued to think about your bad situation with your boss over and over, it could have the potential to ruin your entire vacation.

This is what happens with chronic pain. Repetitive negative thoughts about your pain—or anything else—produce anxiety and create neurological circuits.

Once the circuits associated with pain are established in your nervous system they cannot be eliminated. It *is* possible to influence your own thoughts, however, and create "detours" around these disconcerting pathways. This is the basis of a branch of psychotherapy called cognitive behavioral therapy (CBT). According to the theory behind CBT you can, through a series of directed exercises, "reprogram" or "re-structure" your thinking and improve your mental health. This is a much different process than striving for positive thinking or "mind over matter." There's no way to outrun chronic pain or these relentless circuits. CBT exercises will be presented in detail in the Chapter 9: Solving Stress, the Homework.

THE NATURAL PROGRESSION OF ANXIETY

Although anxiety starts with a thought that causes a reaction, there is a step in between. A negative thought sparks an image, which then elicits the reflexive anxiety response. This happens because the circuits etched into our minds include images as well as thoughts. The imagery involved can be especially compelling and/or disruptive but it occurs so quickly that you usually aren't aware of its role.

According to David Burns, the thoughts and images we are considering here are usually based on cognitive distortions—called "errors in thinking"—which then lead to the development of "stories."[1]

A story is a preoccupation about some aspect of yourself or circumstance of your life that you think is negative, and often includes self-judgment. Typically, the story becomes so entrenched that you're convinced it can't be changed, such as "I can't communicate well," "I'm a disorganized person," or "I'm bad at relationships." Or it can be about an event that caused you stress: "The doctor did the wrong surgery."

A friend of mine once started judging himself about his golf game. He became convinced that he just "couldn't play anymore." As I watched him play, his game seemed pretty much the same to me. He had developed one or two small swing flaws that added a couple strokes to his score, but instead of putting these flaws in perspective, every bad shot confirmed in his mind that he was playing badly. Whenever he hit a good shot, which was fairly frequently, he thought it was luck. If he'd taken a couple of simple lessons he very likely could've improved his game. Instead, he eventually quit playing golf altogether.

In another example from my own experience, I knew a guy who was going through a series of failed relationships. He became discouraged and decided that he "wasn't good at relationships." Every encounter became something that reinforced this story. Instead of working on developing some better skills in this area, he just gave up. He also became chronically frustrated, which did not improve his situation. Regardless of any physical or social attributes one might possess, anger is not attractive.

The problem is a little more serious than it would appear on the surface. That's because the story that's in your head at any given moment becomes your reality.

An example of a story that morphed into reality occurred one day when I was skiing with one of my son's best friends, Holt, who is essentially part of our family. We were out on a fantastic day in Park City, Utah. My son, Nick, had taken off to practice jumping for his mogul competition. Holt and I were relaxing on the chairlift, but he was not in a great mood. When I asked him what was going on, he told me about an incident that had happened the night before.

A friend of his was being harassed in a bar and when he walked over to see what he could do to help, he got physically thrown out. It was bad enough that the bouncer was acting irrationally, but even worse, the local police had also taken quick action without asking any questions. As we talked, I pointed out to him that he wasn't really skiing with me; he was so caught up in the story of what had happened that he was still back in the bar. Although his frustrations were justified, he was allowing people he didn't like take away his ability to enjoy a rare opportunity for us to be able to ski together. It was enlightening to watch him go through a little process of acknowledging what was going on and then truly let it go. I could see how the leftover imagery in Holt's head had been his reality at that moment which gave me a deeper perspective on how this sequence occurs.

We also talked about his choices. I had read William Glasser's book, *Choice Theory,*[2] a few months earlier. It's an excellent book about how to effectively relate to adverse circumstances. One choice would be to change the circumstances. If you don't have that choice, though, you can change how you relate to them. In Holt's situation he was bringing the situation from the night before to a beautiful ski day. After I pointed this out, he made the choice to find out the name of the policeman on the case and either deal with it or drop it, and then he could make the choice to enjoy his day. The choice he did not make—which is critical—was to suppress his frustration and *then* try to enjoy the day. If he had taken that route, those thoughts that had become a story complete with imagery would eventually have surfaced and somehow come out as irrational behavior. It was also interesting to both of us that although we'd talked about these concepts for a couple of years, this situation really brought them home. We ended up having a great time for the rest of the day.

The stories we develop about ourselves and our lives can be deadly to our mental health because we start to interpret random events in a biased way. Many people develop a personal story about their life, casting themselves in a certain role, and then play that role over and over, leaving very little room for wonder and creativity.

With stories about our chronic pain, the stakes are even higher. This is because often the events that started you on your path to pain are disturbing in themselves. Once this is added to an unpleasant physical sensation—which intensifies the repetition of every detail—it's not unlikely that the rest of your bad luck in life will get blamed on those circumstances, whether they're related or not.

One of my chronic pain patients, a fifty-year-old man, had been hit head-on by a drunk driver in a semi-truck. His major injuries had healed but he was still suffering from severe low back pain. Although the accident had occurred five years earlier, he talked about it like it happened yesterday. It had become the central story of his life. He had given up control of his existence to the negligent truck driver.

What are your stories? What imagery do you have in your mind about yourself, your family, spouse, work, and so on?

Cinema Paradiso

A great movie that captures the effects of holding onto "stories" is *Cinema Paradiso*, which won the Oscar for best foreign film in 1989. The film also explores the power of imagery. I suggest watching it (the shorter version) to get a deeper sense of the role stories and imagery play in our lives. For me, this movie had several important messages:

- The mind works in images that are extremely powerful.
- The mind doesn't work in terms of time. If you're holding on to the person or situation that "destroyed your life," which becomes your life's "story," it probably seems like it just happened yesterday. What does happen over time, though, is that the images associated with this story will be reinforced and become stronger.
- Imagery is one of the reasons why an intense negative experience continues to have long-term effects on your sense of well-being. Your story seems like your reality. Time does not always heal if you're not using tools to "let it go." (Note, convincing yourself that you have

let go of your past by suppressing it is the worst choice you can make, for reasons I've already outlined).

- Imagery is why you can see an old close friend you haven't seen for many years and it seems like you saw them just yesterday.
- Imagery can also be used in a powerfully constructive fashion, which is encouraging.

SOCIETAL REINFORCEMENT OF ANXIETY

We've established that thoughts awaken or produce images that cause the body to respond reflexively. Consider how imagery is used all around us to induce anxiety, which influences our behavior.

Marketing

The marketing world has a major impact on our anxiety. A marketer's goal is to produce images of what we should own, look like, or experience in order to be happy and fulfilled. The more subtle (or not-so-subtle) message is that we are less than adequate humans if we don't possess the things they want us to buy. In other words, if we feel badly enough about ourselves, we'll take action in the form of purchasing goods or experiences to decrease our anxiety. In this day and age, we are constantly exposed to intense marketing imagery. It's impossible to escape it without becoming a recluse.

Just consider the body image problem. Eating disorders are epidemic. In a 2004 study out of Norway almost one in five females experienced an eating disorder, and this is also becoming a male issue.[3] Men have historically taken a different tack in the form of aggressive bodybuilding. I remember in seventh grade being ecstatic when my parents bought me a set of weights so I could transform my scarecrow frame. Didn't work. These days obesity is at an epidemic level for both genders. There are many causes, but I think one central factor is the negative cycle of feeling anxious about not having the body you want and the difficulty of achieving one's ideal. The emotional energy you might use to go and exercise, organize your diet, etc. gets burned up in a cycle of anxiety and frustration.

There is so much anxiety in our society created by not feeling good about one's body: think of the industries based on solving the problem with diets, exercise programs, makeup, clothes, or plastic surgery. The list is endless. If the anxiety could be more successfully tolerated, the need for these products and services would rapidly diminish.

The imagery presented to us in the media has always been unattainable by most of us. Now, with digital touching up of photos, even the models themselves cannot attain what's being presented as ideal to the masses.

The resultant problem is twofold. The media imagery becomes more intense over time, both with marketing techniques and in our minds, and we become less equipped to resist it. It becomes increasingly difficult to actually live and enjoy your life.

Familial Imprinting

During the first ten to twelve years of your life, your immediate environment is downloaded into your brain. At that age, you have little ability to edit and interpret. Then, as you get older, you use that database to create a life that is fulfilling and productive. Even the most perfect family situation causes us to download data that's flawed. While it's a common belief that many mental health problems have a genetic basis, the early programming of the brain is a significant factor.

In 1960, a man named Robert Hoffman conceived a concept he termed the "Negative Love Syndrome."[4] In the Negative Love Syndrome, a child instinctively adopts most if not all of his parents' behavioral patterns in order to be accepted and loved. It's both an emotional and physical survival tool. Hoffman started a program called the Hoffman Process, in which participants learn how to become aware of these patterns. The first step is to identify the dysfunctional patterns of each parent; next, you identify your own. Before doing the Hoffman Process I'd spent many years working on myself and was shocked to find out how many of these patterns were controlling my life.

This eight-day in-house program is designed to give you the tools to recognize and process these patterns so they no longer run your life. It allowed me to connect to my own personal value system and to separate myself from my background on a certain level. This is an example of the "reprogramming" concept that we discussed earlier in the chapter.

Anxiety in its many forms is a predominant pattern that's passed on to us from our families of origin. Any time you feel anxiety you are in a pre-programmed pattern. The Hoffman tools allow you to choose your response to any given situation instead of having a predictable, unmediated response.

The Hoffman Process also dramatically organized my thinking in a way that allowed me to write this book. I will discuss its methods more in detail in the "Homework" chapter.

Cultural Programming

I am not going to spend a lot of time on this one; it's an extraordinarily frustrating topic for me to even consider. Throughout world history, rulers have controlled populations by fear. The bully we all feared and hated in school is often in charge. Released from the constraints of adolescence, these rulers typically come to power using the same techniques they employed on the playground.

How often in history has the most competent person been the leader? Is there any training required to become a dictator other than the ruthless use of power? Somehow the human race can't seem to change that paradigm.

A big difference between schoolyard days and adulthood is that the people in charge use visually brutal tactics to subjugate the population. This really hit me the other day when I was reading about a statesman in the 1500s who accompanied his ruler to observe the systematic torture of a population who had attempted an uprising. Torture is also used by gangs to keep their "soldiers" in line. What happens to anyone who resists? The consequences are extremely disturbing, both visually and emotionally. Millions of women underwent trial by torture to determine if they were witches by the Catholic church over hundreds of years. Why were heretics so brutally tortured? The list of gruesome acts is endless and still ongoing. And in this day and age of the Internet we are all even more connected to atrocities and images of them. Much if not most of the world's population is *still* controlled by fear.

I feel incredibly fortunate to live in a country where civil rights have such a high priority. I have the luxury of being able to write this book about anxiety and have the chance to process this emotion. If I lived under a totalitarian regime, I don't think I would have much insight into processing anxiety; instead, I would be controlled by it. Is there a certain level of cultural anxiety that is impossible to rise above? I think so. If you are fortunate enough to escape from the situation, does it leave a permanent scar? Obviously, the answer is yes. However, once you have escaped, you do have the choice of recognizing the depth of the scar and moving forward.

The fear that is used to control of most of the world factors deeply into how our brains are programmed. It's reinforced by world events such as the Great Depression, the two World Wars, 9/11, etc. The impact of these events can last a lifetime. My parents' behavior was permanently affected by their experience of being raised in the Depression era.

The world's religions are at least partly based on the fear of death, which is our ultimate fear. Almost all organized religions use vivid imagery and repetition to imbed a basic set of beliefs aimed at quelling this fear. It's a very effective method—which you could also call a programming process—and adherents of rigid belief systems usually have little fear of death. Unfortunately, it also allows people to be controlled by the institution that is the source of the dogma.

Our parents do imprint upon us positive, loving patterns, but negative behaviors and attitudes are also passed down. Unfortunately, as life progresses there is more reinforcement of the negative patterns. Life generally does not get easier as we move through it.

THE MYTH OF SELF-ESTEEM

Self-esteem is one of the worst concepts ever propagated in the human experience. It implies that if you have enough of "X" then you'll have less anxiety, less frustration, and more happiness. "X" can be material, physical, experiential, relationship-oriented, or almost anything.

Self-esteem is a subtle form of masking. Building self-esteem doesn't help you get rid of anxiety or anger, it only covers them up. Self-esteem blocks the entire goal of the reprogramming process, which is to process anxiety by becoming aware of its effect on your quality of life.

As we talked about in Chapter 3, using self-esteem to lessen anxiety is impossible. Why? For one thing, it's been estimated that the "emotional brain" is four hundred times more powerful than the "rational brain." Clearly, it's an unfair matchup. You can't successfully deal with the irrational pathways of anxiety with rational thinking alone.

Self-esteem actually worsens your anxiety levels: when you've reached the "pinnacle" of scoring achievements and gaining possessions but you're still suffering from anxiety, *then* where do you go? What do you do next? You are now really frustrated.

Our society has taken the cult of self-esteem even further. We're so focused on winning that many of us cease to really enjoy the experience or the activity at hand. Winning is fine, but remember, only a small percent of individuals can win in any given scenario.

I've seen the downside of focusing on winning via my son Nick and his friend Holt, who are world-class mogul skiers. During training, both were so (understandably) set on clinching first place that it compromised their day-to-day enjoyment of the activity itself. I often spoke to both of them about how winning an Olympic medal or a national championship wouldn't have much impact on their lives in the long run; it was more important to appreciate and enjoy the whole act of competing.

In 2007, Holt won the national championship in mogul skiing, an achievement he readily attributes, at least in part, to the awareness and visualization techniques presented in this book. Much of his success, he said, was due to letting go of the outcome and performing with freedom. The more focused he was on winning, the less consistent his performance was. The day after his victory he turned to his performance coach David Elaimy and me and said, "You were right. Winning changed my life for about twelve hours. Life moves on."

It's excellent to strive for excellence and be a productive human being, but it has nothing to do with decreasing your anxiety and frustrations.

Self-esteem involves self-judgment. Judgment, whether it's positive or negative, directed at yourself or others, is one step removed from being fully aware of what's immediately in front of you.

If I seem a little touchy about this subject, I am. I have seen numerous colleagues and friends who were "living the dream" fall into such deep despair that they committed suicide. They had education, money, big reputations, and beautiful families, and yet it didn't make a difference in the end. This list includes four out of eighty of my medical school classmates, two close friends, and twelve additional medical colleagues. These men and women had enough achievements and possessions to ensure self-esteem, and yet the anxious, perfectionist drive that pushed them to the top also destroyed them.

I believe that often people don't kill themselves because they are depressed, they kill themselves because they are anxious. They eventually fold under intense, relentless, progressive anxiety. When you can no longer control the anxiety, anger ensues.

Suicide is in many cases an angry, aggressive act that becomes the only escape from extreme anxiety.

If you are connected with who you are today, you can create the life you want. If you are creating a life to fill a hole inside you, that's a major problem.

THE LIFETIME PROGRESSION OF ANXIETY

Untreated anxiety will always progress. I can't make that point strongly enough. The natural progression of anxiety is:

- Normal situation-appropriate anxiety response
- Generalized anxiety disorder
- Panic disorder
  - Anxiety-based reactions
  - Panic attacks
- Obsessive-compulsive disorder
- Schizophrenia? (This is my own theory and not necessarily supported by the mental health community. But that is a topic for another book.)

Using just a one-word progression, the sequence would go like this:

- Nervous/anxious
- Worried
- Fearful
- Panicked
- Terrified

The tragedy of the progression of anxiety is that it's also eminently treatable. When I say "treatable," I'm not referring to treating the symptoms of anxiety. Rather, I'm talking about using tools to "break up" the related neurologic circuits and halt the progression. You can learn to live with anxiety instead of having it run your life.

Common Ways of Halting the Progression

I feel there is an inherent sense in all of us that if we do not do adequately cope with anxiety, we somehow will lose our minds. Some of the coping mechanisms we use are:

- Suppression/denial
- Rigid/structured thinking
- Avoiding anxiety-producing situations
  - Phobias
  - Decreasing the "size" of your life
- Masking
  - Addictions
  - Distractions
- Pursuit of power
  - Ways to gain more power
  - Gain strength
    ~ Physical
    ~ Mental
    ~ Spiritual
    ~ Financial
- Control
  - People
    ~ Marry, have kids, have complete control of the household
    ~ Employer/employee
  - Circumstances

What percent of successful people are driven by anxiety, and mask it, instead of being driven by a vision based on love?

Many of the above endeavors are worthwhile and greatly contribute to one's quality of life and the welfare of society. However, if the drive to pursue them is anxiety-based instead of love-based, then the consequences can be significant. Many people use these strategies and manage not to be crippled by anxiety, but it always catches up with you in the long run.

Mind you, many of us have little coping methods that do not interrupt our lives. For instance, a businesswoman friend of mine once asked me to dinner specifically to discuss her own tactics in light of the stress management concepts that I teach. She was curious because while she was not experiencing much anxiety, she did have certain habits, like brushing her teeth a specific way and doing counting rituals. She was aware that her behavior was a little odd. After talking to her for a while, I realized that she was living a pretty reasonable life. Her self-owned business was quite successful but purposefully kept small. Her strategies for keeping anxiety at bay were working. From my point of view, it didn't look like she needed to make any significant changes or embark on new endeavors.

Many coping strategies do work. However, I assume that if you are reading this book, then the elephant still in the room is the fact that you are experiencing pain and your life is not as fulfilling and happy as you would like.

I not uncommonly have patients who are in crippling, severe pain, are completely disabled, and yet rank themselves as a zero on the anxiety, depression, and irritability scales on my spine intake questionnaire. Their anxiety-suppressing mechanisms have worked: they are disconnected from their own anxiety. But you can't be disconnected from your anxiety and be connected to yourself.

SUMMARY

The intent of this chapter is to have you look at anxiety from a different perspective. Many people adopt coping strategies without having any idea that they're reacting to a life based on fear. Creating an awareness of how anxiety affects you is the first step to managing it effectively.

The best ways to decrease anxiety and its hold on you are much different than what you may have been taught. My goal is to show you specific reprogramming tools so you can apply them to your life.

Anxiety is a universal, normal part of the human experience. You cannot get rid of it. The key is to understand how to process it effectively so that it does not control your life.

In the next two chapters, we'll discuss anger and how it markedly magnifies anxiety-producing neurologic circuits.

CHAPTER 5

Anger/Victimhood

A major antidote to anxiety is the feeling that
you're in control. Loss of control leads to anger.
In other words, we respond to anxiety by trying to control
the circumstances that cause it, whether it's a situation, person,
or just thoughts. If we can't control these, anger strikes. Anger
boosts your efforts to gain control of your anxiety and helps
you to cover up the feeling. This is what happens when you're
in chronic pain. Your life has been completely disrupted and
you don't know if the pain will ever stop. It may be hard to
go to work or even to get out of bed. You feel like you've lost
control of the ability to influence your own situation, which
would make anyone angry. As with anxiety, though, it's crucial
to understand your anger and process it in a healthy way.
Unprocessed anger weakens your mental health and leads to a
vicious cycle that will intensify your pain.

Anger is an understandable response to chronic pain. You may
find yourself angry for some or all of the following reasons:

- You can't escape the pain—you feel like a victim and
  you are a victim.

- The medical system has no answer for why you're in pain, nor any definite prescription for improvement.
- Your irritability is making your relationships suffer; instead of being an energy source for your family, you are a drain on them.
- You're on disability leave, but your employer and insurance company impatiently pressure you to return to work.
- You often can't get approval for reasonable care. The disability system increases your stress, and yet often won't allow access to resources that would help you deal with it.

How can you not be angry? You have lost control of almost every aspect of your existence. But anger, no matter how justified, will destroy your quality of life.

VICTIMHOOD

In my experience, to become angry you must first feel like a victim. The sequence is:

- Circumstance (perceived or real)
- Blame
- Victim
- Frustration/Anger

Let's look at how it unfolds. First, you blame a person or circumstance for disrupting your sense of well-being, which automatically puts you in the role of a victim. Feeling that you've been the victim of something or someone causes frustration and anger.

The blame-victim-anger sequence can start with either a perceived wrong or an actual wrong. When it's a perceived wrong it's easy to be misled by your thought process. Your mind creates a story about the event, but there's a good chance that the triggering event wasn't a "real" wrong. Examples include being cut off in traffic or being inadvertently left off a party list. Even if it was a random act, you feel victimized. Whatever thoughts or imagery exist in your mind create your version of reality and you are angry about it.

In the second case, you have genuinely been wronged. Someone robbed you. You had surgery that ended up with a severe complication. A driver ran a red light and totaled your car. Here, you *are* a victim in the truest sense. Being in chronic pain is real victimhood.

Whether the victim role is just perceived or actual, the anger response will be exactly the same. The imagery in your mind from the perceived wrong will elicit as strong a response as being treated badly, so both scenarios are equally destructive to your mental health. The difference is that when you actually are a victim it's much harder to let that role go. This puts you at a disadvantage, because you cannot experience the full benefit of forgiveness until you forgive the person who has wronged you the most.

Playing the victim is a universal part of the human experience, since none of us has complete freedom of action. This is particularly true in the context of chronic pain. We are limited by:

- Basic human needs (eating, drinking, sleeping, breathing, etc.)
- Money
- Time
- Physical attributes and conditions (appearance, intelligence, abilities)
- Opportunity

It's how you relate to your limitations, including chronic pain, that determines whether you feel like a victim or not.

There are some people who resist playing the victim even under extreme circumstances. For example, consider the life of

Nelson Mandela. Unjustly imprisoned for twenty-five years, he forgave his captors and went on to become a gracious states-man. He even put some of his former captors to work in his security force.

An almost incomprehensible story is that of Victor Frankel, a Jewish Austrian psychiatrist who survived the World War II concentration camps. At one point he was slated to undergo human medical experimentation. Instead of going into the victim role, he asked himself the question, "What is life asking of me right now?"[1]

I once had a patient who suffered a terrible complication after a major spine operation, one that resulted in permanent blind-ness. Somehow the blood supply to the optic nerve had been compromised during the procedure. Everyone was shocked, as the surgery had initially seemed to go so well. About three months later he walked into my office and said to me, "This is the hand I've been dealt. I'm going to play it." I saw him again eight years later to remove his spinal implants. He was still completely blind, had gone through a bitter divorce, and had experienced several significant financial setbacks. However, he still had the same proactive mindset.

I personally play the victim as well as anyone. However, I have a strong commitment to myself and to my family to recognize and then stay out of that role. Recognition is the first step.

It's Not Them—It's You!!

The most difficult part of understanding anger is acknowledg-ing that it's not the other person or the situation that's causing you to become angry, it's you. Every bit of it. All another person or situation does is trigger a neurological response within you. Robert Hoffman (co-developer of the Hoffman Process) used the psychological term "transference" for this phenomenon.[2] No one can *make* you angry; you have a choice every time your anger button is pushed. The problem is that it doesn't *feel* like you have a choice because the transference response is so fast and powerful. It gives you a strong conviction of your "rightness." Sudden action is often taken while under the spell of transference; it's a dangerous situation. Fortunately, though, transference isn't lasting. Have you ever noticed how quickly the feeling disappears once its runs its course?

Recognizing and acknowledging that my anger response is *my* issue and not the other person's is far and away my own biggest personal challenge. Looking back on my life, I see that anger has been the single greatest factor in my taking abrupt and impulsive actions that have been self-destructive and destructive to my relationships. For me, it has historically been a huge energy drain. Even though I have become much more in touch with my emotions over time, I know that my anger-based responses are still very deep and are not going to disappear. As I write this chapter, I still tend to feel "right" in any conflict and continue to blame a given person or circumstance that upsets me in any given scenario. However, I now see that I'm experiencing transference and try not to take any action until I've used the tools I've been given to defuse my anger. As soon as I "wake up," I'm always amazed how temporarily disconnected I was from the actual situation in question. It really is a state of temporary insanity.

I did not comprehend the devastating power of anger in my life until I participated in the in-house eight-day Hoffman process in Napa Valley. I have mentioned this process before. It was there that I realized that my baseline state of being was "disguised anger."

Hoffman's Definition of Transference

"Transference distorts relationships. Transference is reacting to and perceiving another person as if they are the mother and father from our childhood. Usually we are not aware that we are doing it. We believe we are really seeing that other person in the present moment. When we are in transference with another person, we often feel a certainty that we know who they are. We usually feel we know what they are feeling and thinking, what their intentions are, and what we can and cannot expect from them.

When we are in negative transference (a much more common occurrence for most of us), we feel the energy of certainty about the other person's wrongness. At times, the transference is triggered by an actual behavior of the other person. They don't look us in the eye, or they do. They criticize our work. They are sarcastic or late or forget to do something. Many times the transference is triggered only by our perception that they did something wrong and our interpretation of what that means. We go into a vicious cycle within ourselves. We feel that something wrong has been done to us by another person. We think we know all about them, what they did, and what they will do, think, and feel. They are powerful—we give them the power to affect our lives—and we are powerless. We often feel little, like a child in the face of a negative parent. That's where we went internally even if we do not recognize it consciously.

Actually we have the power, if we choose to use it, to change the dynamic, to stop reacting. The actions of others trigger us because we have the patterns in us." [3]

Waking Up to My Own Victim Role

I lived much of my life as a true victim, although I was unaware of it until age fifty. I was raised in an abusive household which was my only reality. It was only through extensive counseling that I realized my childhood was not the norm. Every mental health professional I encountered pointed out that the abuse I endured was severe.

Of course, I don't have the corner on suffering. Truthfully, I thought my family story was somewhat unusual until I attended an event in connection with Hyde School, where my daughter went for her junior and senior years of high school. Located in Bath, Maine, the school is unique in that the founder, Joey Gauld, has made character development the school's highest priority. It also offers an excellent academic program in addition to the arts and athletics. The students meet regularly and challenge each other to reach for their individual potential. Three times each year the families also take part in group meetings.

At my first Joey Gauld seminar in 2007, I was in a large circle with about twenty other parents. He asked the question, "What problems do you think that your family passed on to you that you may have passed on to your child?" and gave each of us five minutes to answer. He was eighty years old at the time and an amazing individual. In five to ten minutes he would assess the issue and give pearls of insight that were priceless.

As we went around the circle, I was shocked to hear that all but one parent had endured various forms of abusive upbringing including neglect, alcoholic rages, emotional and physical abuse, etc. It was interesting to note that every parent in the circle had a successful career. Whether they were CEOs of huge corporations or working in a smaller arena, it did not matter. The stories were dismal. Only then did I realize that sharing my personal struggles under the guise of "helping" others was yet another way of remaining in the victim role. Five years after I had "given up" the victim role, I was still deeply in it. Life is a humbling experience.

My history of abuse had a powerful effect on my life and by 2002, five years before the Gould seminar, I had been in a terrible emotional state. I could barely make it through the day. I remained a technically excellent surgeon but internally I was miserable. I was experiencing severe burnout and had pursued every possible avenue of help with a vengeance, but nothing seemed to work. In fact I was getting progressively worse.

A crucial turning point came for me in May of 2002 while I was outside with my future wife and daughter washing their car. It was a beautiful Mother's Day and I had every reason to feel happy. But instead of being happy, I was in mental agony, enveloped in anxiety. This juxtaposition of the lovely day and my misery made no sense. I started thinking about how tired I was of all my internal unrest. Then all of a sudden, I realized how much I had placed myself in the victim role. It hit me like a lightning bolt. That moment led me to a deep decision, one that would eventually pull me out of my despair: I would stop playing the victim. The sequence of events that brought me to that decision was complex, but the decision itself was simple. Within six weeks my anger began to abate. Three months later, I had made major changes in my life.

It took another year before I really pulled out of my tailspin, but my life took a crucial turn that weekend. One of the realizations I came to was that I'd been on an endless pilgrimage to find the one answer that would change things and relieve my suffering. I'd been searching for an outside source to solve my problem, continually looking to be fixed or find a way to fix myself. But one day I realized that there *was* no one simple answer. Instead, it was to be an ongoing process without an endpoint—I was, and would be, continually evolving.

Then I returned to David Burns' book *Feeling Good*.[4] The cognitive behavioral therapy in the book had had a major impact on me in the past, but I'd given it up. By not pursuing a resource that I knew was powerful I was essentially choosing to remain a victim. At that point I wasn't aware of how to develop alternative neurological pathways—all I knew was that the book's exercises worked for me. Plus, I noted that the author said that the book's cognitive restructuring was effective in relieving anxiety 85% of the time. I re-committed to Burn's writing and repetition techniques.

Years after I started the *Feeling Good* exercises, the Hoffman Process added a major dimension to my understanding of the role anger played in my life. These two resources have been pivotal in transforming that life.

The Disguises of Anger

There are many creative ways to be a victim. There are also many ways to hide it both from others and from yourself. None of us like the idea that we might be playing the victim role and so we tend to disguise it. The list of disguising methods is infinite, but here are a few common ones:

- Having strong opinions
- Feeling sorry for yourself
- Suppressing your negative thoughts
- Dissociating—closing the door on the past
- Adopting an identity of being "cool and calm"
- Being perfectionistic and judgmental

As you become more honest with yourself and recognize your victimhood, you can at least give yourself a little credit for creativity. I joke with my patients that disguising my anger is my most highly developed life skill. I wish it was a just a joke.

When I think about being a victim, one day I spent with my wife sticks out in my mind. It's a good example of how the "poor me" mode can set in quickly and negatively affect what could otherwise be a great day.

It happened when my wife and I went hiking in Yosemite. I will preface this story by letting you know that my wife is a true city girl. She is the only person I know who would go hiking with me in high-heeled sneakers and a mini-skirt. Although she lived in the Bay area, only about four hours drive away, she'd never been to the park. She was very concerned about the bears and all of the bear warning signs did not help to allay her anxiety. I had been going to Yosemite for years and earnestly assured her that bears weren't very active during the day and were therefore not going to be a problem.

On our hike we met a couple of women at the Vernal Falls bridge. One of them was an avid nature photographer and excitedly told us how she had seen three bears in the last two days. Of course in that moment I lost all credibility with my wife.

Two days later, we were leaving the Awanhee Hotel on the floor of the valley on what couldn't have been a more clear or beautiful day. The road to Glacier Point had just opened and there were very few people around. As we got into the car, my wife made a comment about the bear warning sign in front of the hotel. From her perspective, her comment was light and a joke. But I took it personally as an assault on my character. Instead of letting it go, I held on to it and stopped talking to her. I was feeling very sorry for myself. The ensuing conversation was one I wouldn't have chosen for such a wonderful drive. I couldn't let go of the fact that "she was the one who started it all" and blamed her for ruining our drive up to that point.

Fortunately, my wife is a little wiser than I in these type of conflicts. She wasn't thrilled with me but talked to me in a way that helped me see that I was playing the victim. I'm thankful for the people in my life, like my wife, who can provide me with a reality check.

I'd like to say that I was never again the source of that kind of tension between my wife and me; however, that's not the case. I do consider these situations to be learning experiences though and try to use them to avoid similar interchanges in the future. Doing so will only affect my relationships and quality of life in a positive way.

A second example of my tendency to victimhood was when I repeatedly told my wife that I needed to write this book but was working too hard and didn't have enough time. I finally realized that I was allowing myself to be a victim of circumstances and the clock. I had three choices. One was to continue to complain and remain agitated. Another was to forget about the book, taking it off of my "to-do list." A third was to write and finish the book. That insight allowed me to realize how much of my energy was being drained by not taking full responsibility for my actions. Hence I am able to share this book with you.

Choosing to Remain a Victim

Being a victim is among the deepest rooted of human behavioral patterns, one that is dramatically reinforced in the presence of chronic pain. It's also a powerful role that works very well. Consider the advantages:

- Others expect less of you
- You expect less of yourself
- You have a feeling of power, which masks the feeling of anxiety
- It gives you a sense of entitlement
- You "justifiably" manipulate those around you
- There is a sense of conviction and being "right"

The workers' compensation system often leads a chronic pain sufferer to embrace a kind of victimhood that is *real* victimhood in the truest sense. In this scenario you are usually treated terribly and have very little control of the circumstances. (If you don't feel angry, then you must be incredibly skilled at suppressing that anger.) The only control you have is to remain in the victim role. If you are angry with your employer, you can really stick it to them with the cost of your medical care. Why get better? No one really seems to care. However, choosing victimhood instead of attempting to get better doesn't really work. Your employer will survive. Your claims examiner will go to work tomorrow. There's not one person you're going to permanently harm. Yet you have allowed chronic anger to erode your quality of life.

The best you can do with this pattern is to recognize when it's interfering with your life. Part of being able to emerge from the victim role is understanding its power and resisting it.

I know that it's hard to commit to a different way of living. We all have familiar patterns, and it makes us anxious if we have to give them up. There's comfort in being a victim. Somehow we are willing to continue to suffer rather than change—the anxiety associated with change may feel worse than remaining in your current circumstances. There are numerous studies done on chronic illness which show that patients drop out of treatment 30-50% of the time. It does not seem to depend on the success of the treatment.[5] If you're hesitant to give up your patterns, know that the discomfort you feel in the process of changing isn't permanent. It will lead you to gaining your life back.

I am well aware of how terrible chronic patients' lives can be due to circumstances that are out of their control. However, they are also allowing their life energies to be drained instead of using them to solve their problems.

Validation

Another major factor in playing the victim role is the need to be validated. This need sneaks up on you and may be much stronger than you can perceive. If there's no identifiable source of pain on a test, patients feel that no one believes their pain is real. I personally believe my patients are in pain; it's just that usually I can't find a definitive source. However they become understandably obsessive about the possibility that something serious has been missed. There's also the issue of when a patient meets with a surgeon who thinks mechanically and whose language revolves around the idea that there *must* be an identifiable injury that's causing the pain.

The patients who need to be validated are my most difficult cases. They are so wrapped up in being "right" that it's difficult to reach them. Sadly, their all-consuming preoccupation has usually made their lives—and the lives of those close to them—miserable.

It has been shown that when patients with chronic abdominal pain end up with a diagnosis of terminal pancreatic cancer, a high percentage of them report a significant improvement in their sense of well-being. The most common reason cited is that once they have an identifiable problem, others will believe their pain is real.

A surgical scar can also be validating, no matter what the outcome of the surgery. In Dr. Peter Fritzell's study looking at patients who had undergone fusion for low back pain versus non-operative care, 16% of the patients who did poorly stated that they would choose to undergo the surgery again.[6] A scar on one's back is a strong justification of suffering.

One patient who came to me wanting surgery many years ago had been in constant low back pain for over four years after being rear-ended in a car accident. Gordon, thirty-two, had undergone two laminectomies before he saw me, both done between the fourth and fifth lumbar vertebrae, but neither had brought him relief. When I saw him I couldn't find an identifiable structural source of his pain and therefore did not recommend any further surgery.

I was determined to get Gordon back on track. At that point, I wasn't yet practicing a fully formed version of the DOCC program, although I did have a good understanding of the effects that stress and lack of sleep have on pain and used those concepts with Gordon.

I saw Gordon every one to two weeks for over eight months. He was under some intense personal stresses and was very anxious. I used several stress reduction techniques with him, all to no avail.

Gordon finally fired me and saw a surgeon in a neighboring town. He had a fusion done at L4-5 both from the front and back of his spine. After the surgery, he not only felt great, he took out an ad in the local paper thanking his new surgeon for doing such an excellent job.

I did not feel good about my experience with Gordon. It's not as if a fusion never works, it's just not predictable enough to warrant it being done in someone so young. I also knew that in five to ten years, there was the chance of his spine breaking down around the fusion—it was something I had seen firsthand in my career. These factors all went into my decision not to move forward with surgery.

Gordon then filed a malpractice lawsuit against me for not performing the surgery that he thought would have helped him. I was quickly cleared but I had to hire an attorney and go before a panel of peers to deal with it. I still would not have done anything differently. I just wish I had known then what I know now about the mental health aspect of chronic pain. Back then I did not understand the sensitization process or how to calm down the nervous system.

The situation was also awkward in that I frequently ran into Gordon while doing business around town. I was surprised when finally, about a year later, he approached me, looked me in the eye, and said, "You were right." Apparently, the pain relief he'd felt right after the surgery hadn't lasted.

How victimized do you feel by your pain and the circumstances surrounding it? How angry are you that no one seems willing to listen to you, believe you, or care about your pain? How attached are you to your victim role? How willing are you to look at whether it's running your life?

The victim role is universal. The willingness to take an honest look at it is not. Asking yourself all the above questions will help you get closer to moving out of this role.

Perfectionism—the Ultimate Victim Role

Perfectionism is an additional—and perhaps less examined—way that people play the victim. Many view perfection as the standard that must be reached in order to be successful. It's held up as a virtue in all aspects of our lives, especially in professional and vocational endeavors. We feel pressure from others to be perfect, and we feel pressure from ourselves.

Perfection does not exist in the human experience, however. The closest thing to perfection I see is in the nature and design of the human body. A living, fully functioning human organism is beyond wonder. But there's even imperfection there, in the form of death.

Since perfection is unattainable, you'll suffer endless anxiety if you try to reach it. You may label yourself a "failure" and look for someone or something to blame. Passionate anger about the injustice of not attaining the perfection you deserve fills or covers up the gap between perfection and reality. You become a victim of being "less than perfect." It is the ultimate in self-flagellation.

In the context of chronic pain, it's particularly important not to expect a return to some perfect ideal. You may not be as active or productive as you were before the pain started, but this shouldn't be a concern. Instead, simply focus on improvement—becoming more functional—one day at a time.

Victimized by Pain

Being a victim of chronic pain is a unique level of victimhood. Not only do you feel wronged, you are also experiencing an often-excruciating physical sensation without knowing if there is an end in sight. You truly are a victim of that pain. The inability to escape pain elicits an intense feeling of victimization.

To understand this concept, consider that each of your body's senses is designed to protect the nervous system. If you're standing in the road and a car is moving toward you, you move out of the way and feel safe. If you smell leaking gas, you get out of the house and feel relief. If you touch a hot stove, you withdraw your hand and avoid a worse burn. You exert your ability to control the movement of your body, protecting yourself in the process. But with chronic pain, you can't take any action to separate yourself from the pain. You have no control. There's nothing you can do to feel safe, or relieved, or lucky for limiting the pain, and this leads to severe anxiety, then anger and even rage.

As discussed, you can decrease your pain by calming down your nervous system. The perception of pain will diminish—often to zero. This usually occurs during the phase of working through your anger issues.

When I first started the DOCC project, I'd tell my patients that the pain wouldn't go away with better management of stress, but it *would* help them cope with the pain better and live a more enjoyable life. If I could not offer them a surgical solution, I wanted to share some stress management tools that I'd learned through my own difficult journey. I was shocked when many—if not most—of my patients would report a significant decrease in their pain after using the tools. Often it would dissipate completely.

Pain is a significant stressor. It is real and you are a legitimate victim. However, your legitimate reaction of chronic anger will destroy your life.

ANGER—THE ABSOLUTE BLOCK TO REGAINING YOUR LIFE

It has become increasingly clear to me that if a given patient engages in the principles outlined in this book they will experience a dramatic decrease in pain and an improved quality of life. The richness of their new life often even exceeds anything they experienced before their pain nightmare. There is no exact roadmap and often other resources fit a given person's needs better than what I have suggested. Whatever method you use, though, the key is to first address anxiety and then anger, and then continue to "shift" your nervous system so that it's operating with a more functional set of circuits. The plan just needs to be somewhat structured and then earnestly implemented over a period of time.

If a patient is engulfed in anger, it's extremely difficult to get him or her to take part in the reprogramming process. Anger is a barrier that prevents them from moving forward, and I've found it nearly impossible to help them dismantle this barrier. This morphs into chronic anger, which becomes your baseline emotional state. And even though you feel it (anger) all the time, you're unable to recognize it.

The problem with anger is that it takes away your ability to listen to another person and step back to truly assess a given situation. The conversation I have with a patient who is "entrenched" typically goes something like this:

"Doctor, you mean to tell me there's nothing wrong with my back? I've been in pain for several years and I know that this pain is not in my head. You must be missing something."

I reply, "The pain you're experiencing isn't imaginary pain nor is it psychological. We know that if we did a functional MRI of your brain right now, the part of your brain that corresponds to your area of pain would light right up. All that matters is what's happening in your brain. We also know that the brain can fire spontaneously without an identifiable source of the pain. It's not that I don't believe you're in pain; I know the pain is real and you are very frustrated about being trapped by it. I know you feel that there's no way out."

I also explain to them that degenerated discs are a normal part of the aging process and that there is no correlation between a degenerated disc and back pain. And I let them know that the surgical success of a fusion for LBP is less than 30% with a significant downside of a failed surgery.

They then say, "I don't want surgery. I just want to be fixed and get my life back."

When I reply that we've had very consistent results following the steps outlined in this book they usually explode and say something like, "I don't want to read a book or anything like that. Just do something to fix my back." They will then starting ranting, and often yelling, that no one will help them, and occasionally they just walk out of the room.

This is a frequent scenario. I would estimate that at least 50% of my patients fall somewhere on this part of the spectrum. They are entrenched in their anger, which prevents them from engaging in effective treatment. Anger is multi-directional and destructive; it's particularly destructive to one's self. When you encounter an angry person it's similar to stepping on a land mine. They have a strong sense of being "right" at all times and an even a stronger sense that everyone else is wrong.

I honestly don't know what to do to break into this mindset. I've tried everything from being confrontational to being incredibly patient. In most cases nothing has worked. In fact, speaking to them at length just makes them more angry. It appears that people who are angry don't like to be convinced to give up their anger. Maybe they just can't hear me.

ONE FINAL WORD ABOUT ANGER

The ultimate paradox of holding on to anger against someone is that instead of pushing them away, you are giving them complete control over your quality of life. My question is, why are you allowing that person or circumstance to have that kind of power?

There's a famous quote by Oscar Wilde: "Always forgive your enemies; nothing annoys them so much."

When you're angry you are reacting to a problem, not solving it. It's necessary to be creative in order to find solutions. The difference between the word "reactive" and the word "creative" is the location of the letter "c." It's easier to be creative if you're fully aware of the variables causing you to be distressed. You must "see" before taking action.

If you're a victim of chronic pain, and you're angry, the best gift you can give yourself is to learn how to recognize your victimhood, process it, and move on!

CHAPTER 6

Anxiety-Fueled Anger, the Highway to Hell

So far, we've talked about the roles that anxiety and anger play in chronic pain. Now let's look at the connection between the two. Anxiety and anger are so closely intertwined that they can't be treated alone. Understanding this interaction is essential to calming your nervous system.

Anxiety and anger are both connected to the survival instinct. Anxiety, as discussed, makes us feel vulnerable and helpless. The survival instinct leads us to mask these emotions with anger, which makes us feel powerful and purposeful instead of helpless.

Anger, however, is not an antidote for anxiety. In addition to masking anxiety, anger also reinforces it. When you're angry, a barrage of irrational thoughts follows. Anger is the turbocharger that gets your negative circuits really spinning. So at the same time that anger covers up the feeling of anxiety, it's also strengthening these anxiety-producing neurological circuits. It's a deadly cycle.

The interaction between anxiety and anger makes treatment a challenge. In order to focus on dealing with your anxiety, you're being asked to give up your anger and victimhood. Without anger to mask your sense of helplessness, however, it's hard to confront your anxiety. Raw anxiety is a very unpleasant feeling; it's what all living creatures have been programmed to avoid. This may be why many people don't confront their anxiety until it's so extreme that it can no longer be contained by either functional or dysfunctional means.

FACING UP TO YOUR ANGER

For years I didn't recognize my anger. With my expertise in suppressing emotions, I fancied myself a very calm, cool, and collected person. In fact, one of my opening lines to my wife when I met her in 2001 was that I was "one of the few people I knew who had really dealt with his anger issues." If either of us could have known the future. Things changed when my personal circumstances got so bad that I came face to face with my underlying rage—I couldn't escape the fact that it was one of my core patterns. I realized that while I'd dealt with my anxiety, anger was still a major factor in my life. What's more, I saw that being angry had been an incredible drain on my energy level.

When I hit my core anger, it was like an oil gusher. It didn't feel good or cathartic in the least. It felt dirty, noxious, and despicable. However it was only by becoming aware of it and addressing it that my life could change. Within six months of confronting my anger (not completely by choice) my thirteen-year battle with anxiety-driven burnout thankfully came to an end. I still frequently fall back into a victim role, but now I have the tools to quickly come out of it. It has been sobering to realize how much of my life I spent in that mindset. Now I feel much more free.

It's not uncommon for people to deny their anger issues. I often have patients who insist that life is great outside of their chronic pain, but anger keeps emerging in comments like, "The doctor did the wrong operation" or "How could I have had so many operations that didn't work?" The emotional tension is clear to me, but they really can't see it. The elephant in the room is that their chronic pain is not compartmentalized—it resonates throughout their lives as a disability accompanied by anxiety, anger, and general unhappiness.

Remember that the anger associated with chronic pain is the result of being a "real" victim of very real pain. That's why it's extremely difficult to let it go. It's crucial, however, to acknowledge the condition and come to terms with it in order to move forward with your recovery. Anxiety's symptoms are more readily apparent and more commonly treated and yet it's necessary to treat *both* emotions. Even if you're able to decrease your anxiety independently, if you're still angry, the anger will magnify whatever anxiety is left.

In dealing with your anxiety and anger, it's best to treat your anxiety first. If you start with anger, the level of anxiety you uncover may seem unbearable. Once your anxiety is at a reasonable level, you can move on to acknowledging and addressing your anger and frustration.

As you progress in learning and using the programming methods in this book that are the most suited to your needs, the relationship between anger and anxiety in your life will become more clear. Truly engaging in the process is difficult but extremely rewarding. It will transform your life.

My Doctor Is Missing Something:
When You Don't Realize You're in Hell

One danger of denying your anger is that you run the risk of making a bad decision about surgery. Consider this scenario: one of the first questions I ask patients in my clinic is, "What exactly are you looking for?" The most common answer I hear is, "I just want to get rid of the pain." The implication is that post-surgery the rest of their life will come together perfectly and be smooth sailing. Really?

As I am a surgeon, most patients look to me for the surgery that will solve their pain problems. If I identify a structural injury that needs to be dealt with, then I'll aggressively go after it surgically and deal with any anger and stress issues later. However, the vast majority of the patients I see do not have an identifiable structural injury that I can solve with surgery.

I love structural injuries (in the context of my practice, that is). There's nothing more satisfying in my life than to be able to take someone who is in severe pain and give them their life back. Likewise, I dislike telling my patients that there's nothing I can offer surgically to relieve their pain. I don't know any surgeon who likes that situation. It makes me feel almost as helpless as my patient does.

However, I find it completely unacceptable to attempt "long-shot surgery." In basketball, the metaphor would be "throwing up a prayer." As we talked about earlier in the book, if there's no distinct structural injury, then surgery has a low-to-zero chance of solving the pain problem. In addition, there's a severe downside to a failed back surgery: it can cause permanent damage and create unsolvable structural issues. Although it took me a few years to learn to say, "No, I cannot surgically help you," it's much better than attempting an operation with poor odds of success.

So when you've been told by a surgeon—who, by the way, gets paid much more for doing surgery than talking about it—that you don't have the option of surgery, what are you going to do?

If you opt for surgery for a non-structural injury, the chances of a good outcome are dismal. By definition, being in chronic pain means that you are under significant stress: most likely, you haven't yet dealt with your anger and the other issues (lack of sleep, frustration, etc.) that contributed to the pain experience. Consider that the odds of a successful spine fusion to relieve low back pain in a situation where a patient is under *minimal* stress are less than 30%.[1] That percentage plummets when the patient is suffering from chronic pain.

However, even after I've explained this scenario to my patients, they still often say they want to give it a try. My strategy is to then reverse the conversation. I point out to them that they have a 70% chance of not doing well with surgery and the downside risk is more predictable than the upside benefit. If at this point they persist, I have to give up and tell them that I just cannot help them at any level. Unfortunately, they won't have to look very far to find a surgeon to do the operation. Surgery is what surgeons are trained to do.

Not having chronic pain is better than having it; I wouldn't try to convince anyone otherwise. However, it's unlikely that your pain is the cause of all of your problems. Patients become convinced that pain is the source of many of their life issues and that getting rid of it will solve everything. But just as winning the lottery often doesn't change people's lives for the better, ridding yourself of pain won't make as much difference as you'd think.

In this situation, you can continue to be angry about your pain; you can continue to obsess about no one caring or helping you. Or you can wake up and do your best with the hand you were dealt.

The risk of not addressing anger issues was clear with Mary, a patient in her mid-thirties who came to me years ago seeking a second surgical opinion. She'd suffered a lifting injury while in the military, and was angry. The lifting had not caused a structural injury and so I didn't think that her injury warranted surgery. There was another particular to her case: Mary's lower back was moderately curved, a condition she'd had since birth. The term for the disorder is congenital scoliosis. While there is a slightly higher chance of low back pain with scoliosis, I still felt strongly that Mary should not have surgery. I reminded her that patients with straight spines experience the same type of pain after a lifting injury. Also, she hadn't fully participated in a conditioning program, which might've improved her situation. I talked to her for over an hour about why she shouldn't have an operation. Mary's situation was potentially drastic in that she had been advised to have seven levels of her spine fused, including her whole lower back and into her lower thoracic spine. But she was determined to go ahead with it.

Mary's post-operative course was difficult. She returned to me two years later in a wheelchair because of ongoing severe low back pain. Although the fusion hadn't completely healed, it was stable. She now had a recommendation to have the weak spot in her fusion surgically repaired.

The success rate of repairing fusions is high. The chances of relieving this patient's pain, however, were almost zero. Unless the weak area of the fusion is unstable, my feeling is that surgery is not warranted. In addition, her pre-operative mental state had markedly deteriorated after two more years of pain. There was nothing that could be done surgically to relieve her suffering.

I saw Mary before I knew much about comprehensive rehabilitation and the importance of calming down the nervous system by addressing anxiety and anger. Her main reason for returning to see me was to undergo yet another operation. She couldn't let go of the idea that surgery was the definitive solution.

This scenario is common in my experience. A patient has ongoing chronic pain and is justifiably angry about the whole situation. A surgeon offers them an option which seems like a way out of a dark situation; it's hard not to pursue that option in light of the idea that surgery is a "definitive solution." With their anger in full gear, patients are rarely thinking clearly and will often pursue options that have a low chance of success. The downside of failed surgery isn't fully comprehended. Then, when a given operation fails, they pursue surgery again and again.

In another case, a man who'd been suffering low back pain for twelve years came to see me. Jim was about forty and was extremely athletic. He'd undergone a major back operation every eighteen to twenty-four months for ten years and was completely disabled by unrelenting low back pain. Despite his history, Jim had no interest in talking to me about anger, pain, or rehab. I never was able to treat him, as he was off to another surgeon who would "fix" him.

How Many Neck Surgeries Will He Have?

Rick, a fifty-year-old patient from Florida, is another example of someone who was convinced he had a structural injury. Disabled with chronic pain over most of his body for several years, he'd sought me out for a second opinion on his neck. He was experiencing at least ten different symptoms: burning, aching, stabbing, and tingling all over, along with bladder urgency, balance problems, and dizziness. Previously, Rick had had a laminectomy of his neck (where the lamina—or the bone over the back of the spinal cord—is removed to relieve pressure). His symptoms seemed to improve for a little while, but within a couple years his condition worsened and in 2009 he had a fusion through the front of his neck between his fifth and sixth vertebrae. Again there was a slight improvement, but two years later he was in my office with crippling pain throughout his whole body.

As I talked to Rick I could see how desperate he was for relief. He wasn't sleeping and his anxiety and frustration were ten on the zero-to-ten scale of my spine intake questionnaire. When I looked at the MRI scan of his neck I could see where the two prior surgeries had been performed, but I also saw that there were no pinched nerves. The alignment and stability of his vertebrae were also fine. Several workups of his brain and the rest of his nervous system came out normal. I couldn't find anything physically wrong with him.

When I explained to Rick that I didn't see a structural problem that was amenable to surgery, he became, understandably, very upset. He was stuck on the idea that the prior surgeries had helped and that I was missing something. It didn't matter what I said or how I explained it to him.

What I did not tell him was that I had also looked at the scans done prior to his previous operations and couldn't find anything there to warrant surgery either. (Telling a patient that he or she did not really need the prior surgery is a very unproductive and unpleasant interaction.) On the first MRI of his neck there were no bone spurs and the spinal cord was completely free. There was no structural problem that could've been corrected by surgery. The scan before the second operation also failed to show anything that would've caused any symptoms.

What's difficult for patients (and physicians) to realize is that the placebo rate for any medical or surgical treatment is between 25-30%.[2] This is not an imaginary improvement; the body really does feel less pain. With the placebo effect, a part of the brain's frontal lobe actually shuts off pain pathways for short periods of time, which can result in long-lasting relief. When it wears off, though, you're back to where you were pre-surgery.

A prior surgery or procedure that was temporarily effective shouldn't affect your current decision-making about your spine. I continue to practice medicine according to the adage: "If I can see it, I can fix it. If I can't see it, I can't correct anything with surgery."

I suggested that Rick take a look at the DOCC website and told him that I'd be happy to explain the whole program to him in as much detail as needed. I did not think I would hear from him again.

Over the next couple of months I was surprised to receive a couple of emails from Rick and had a telephone conversation with him that seemed to go pretty well. He was willing to engage in the DOCC program and subsequently began some of the writing exercises. Our second talk on the phone a couple of weeks later seemed to go even better, and he said he could see that thinking I'd missed something was part of an obsessive thought pattern. I was encouraged and thought that maybe I'd been able to break through his "story."

Our final conversation, however, was dismal. He had reverted back to his original stance and couldn't let go, after all, of the feeling that a structural problem was being overlooked. He was absolutely positive that his C7 was "out of alignment." I assured him once again that we'd done a thorough check and that as a surgeon I'm quite obsessive about not overlooking anything I can fix. At this point it didn't matter, though—he'd found a surgeon who was going to fuse his neck.

I don't know how many tests and surgeries Rick will undergo over the next thirty years, but I do know that the personal cost to him and to society will be enormous.

What's puzzling to me is that if medical board examiners had looked at the indications for surgery submitted by any of the surgeons who operated on essentially normal anatomy, those surgeons would've been failed immediately for giving a "dangerous answer."

Why Don't You Know You're in Hell?

As a physician, I place a high importance on being able to relate to my patients; only then can I offer them the best quality care. That's why it's frustrating when I feel there's a breakdown in communication in my office consultations. I used to react negatively at patients' seeming inability to understand why lack of a structural injury means they don't need surgery, only to have them ask again why surgery isn't an option. Now, however, I get it.

I've come to understand that my patients' anger over their chronic pain prevents them from seeing anything clearly. Physicians use the term "injury conviction" to describe this phenomenon. It's the relentless pursuit of a cause well beyond reason. My perception of this concept has changed in that I feel that this pattern of thinking becomes its own irrational neurological circuit. Patients are so wrapped up in their own needs that rational arguments have absolutely no effect. Their neurological circuit of anger that's continually triggered by their pain makes them unable to understand and accept the logical conclusion that surgery won't help them.

I still have some difficulty in emotionally grasping this concept, but it's become clearer to me over the years as I see it again and again. I've learned that the thoughts "The doctor is missing something" or "There must be a reason I'm in pain" are circuits that spin independently of any explanation. It's the only reason I can think of that a given patient would go back for more and more surgeries when none of the prior ones were successful. Often they continue to stick with the same surgeon who performed all of the previous failed surgeries. This irrational decision-making is a scenario that the medical profession doesn't fully recognize. I don't know what percentage of major spine surgery decisions are made in this context, but it's safe to say that it's a significant number.

As we discussed in Chapter 5, ingrained neurological circuits can stop you from being able to effectively take part in the many facets of the DOCC program.

THE ABYSS

Patients in chronic pain fall into a certain mental state over time—I call it "the Abyss." The "equation" for the Abyss is the following:

Abyss = (Anxiety x Anger) x Time

In the Abyss, you have lost control of almost everything, including:

- Pain
- Finances
- The ability to be physically active without limitations
- The ability to enjoy anything you do in your spare time without the experience being marred by pain

Other details of the experience include:

- People don't believe you're in pain. Often, the harder you try to convince your friends, family, peers, employers, and health care providers, the less you are believed.
- You're at the mercy of a claims manager who has little medical training and no concept of how your life is being affected by your pain.
- You may have undergone a failed operation or series of operations. You are angry about the outcome and the events that led you to decide to have the surgery in the first place, but you cannot go back.

Then multiply this whole scenario by time, and I think you can begin to understand my point. Not only is there the repetition of anxiety, pain, and frustration, but usually there is no end point and no hope of escape. In some ways it's worse than having the diagnosis of terminal cancer. At least with cancer, people believe you and, for better or for worse, the ordeal will come to an end.

To me, the chronic pain situation is like having your soul pounded into the ground by a pile driver. Your life is being systematically destroyed. What I also find extremely ironic is that you may have achieved a full and successful life only to have it unexpectedly consumed by pain. You had not anticipated this possibility.

The dark place that develops in your mind is often deep. My patients cannot find words to describe the depth of frustration they feel being in the Abyss.

Patients in the Abyss have complained to my staff and administration that I am inconsiderate because I don't believe them and won't perform the surgery they need. I've discovered that the longer I spend talking to them the more likely they are to become upset.

If you're in this group, you really are in hell and I don't know how to help you out of it. May God help you, because I cannot. You are extremely angry and anger is a block not only to your care but also to life itself.

The only way out of the Abyss is through you. If you don't realize you're there, you will remain there. When working with patients in the Abyss, I have learned to let go when I cannot penetrate that firewall of denial. If you have lifted yourself out of this hole, I'd very much like to know what gave you the insight to move forward.

It has been said that anger is temporary insanity. "Temporary" implies that there's hope. If and when you are ready to face up to your anger, I'm always willing to do what I can, even if you were the one who filed a complaint.

Your Family Is Probably in Hell with You:
Pain = Anger = Abuse

Like many professionals I know, I was raised in an abusive household. My mother was physically and emotionally abusive (and she also suffered from chronic pain). It was confusing for me to feel one moment like I had a mother who would do anything for her family and then, the next moment, watch her fly into a rage that could last for several days. From a young child's perspective it was terrifying.

I read a book during my late teens that shed some light on my mother's behavior. It is a brilliant book by Scott Peck called *People of the Lie*. He begins with a story of a twelve-year-old boy who had a near-psychotic break after he was given a 22-caliber rifle for Christmas. His parents were confused in that they felt that they were making a positive statement to him: he was entering his teen years and they trusted him enough to believe he could be responsible with a gun. The problem was that it was the same gun that his fifteen-year-old brother had used to commit suicide the prior Christmas. These parents, like my mother, were unaware of their child's needs.

Being unaware of another person's needs is the essence of abuse. Unfortunately, if you are in chronic pain you run the risk of being abusive to others. If you are consumed by anxiety and trying to keep your head above water, you may well become fixated on your own needs and unable to view a given situation through another person's eyes.

Then take it a step further with regards to anger. When you are angry you cannot see anything clearly; it is truly all about you. What's more, anger is temporary insanity and it's dangerous to interact with people or make decisions in that state of mind. When you're experiencing chronic pain you are frustrated and angry much of the time. You may have a legitimate gripe in that your basic need to be pain-free is not being met. You feel the world, including your family, owes you something. You feel justified in venting your anger, whether it's directed at someone in particular or just expressed to the world at large.

But how do you think your children or partner perceive your mood and actions? How much control do you think a five-year-old feels he has when you're angry or maybe even in a rage after yet again being disappointed by the medical world or beaten up by the worker's comp system? You may not perceive your actions as abusive, but I can guarantee you it's abuse.

I now request that my patients, as part of their healing process, ask their family what it's like to be around them when they're upset and then visualize that scenario from the receiving party's eyes. When they describe what they see, it's not pretty.

I also request that my patients never talk to members of their family when they are upset. They have to go to another room or leave the house, and cannot re-engage until they've calmed down. You cannot suppress or control anger, but you don't have to become a living weapon. Anger can be dealt with using reprogramming strategies.

Wake up!! There are 116 million people in the U.S. suffering from chronic pain. That is one in three. If you consider the effect that pain has on family members, the number of people affected has to be well over half of the population.

MY PLEA

The main predictor of success with the DOCC program is my patients' willingness to be open to change, and then to fully engage. The greater the degree of commitment to the program, the faster the improvement in pain and quality of life; if you spend enough time and effort, success is not a matter of "if," but "when."

Unfortunately, in my experience, for many patients the same anxiety-fueled anger that drove them into the Abyss is what blocks their openness to helping themselves. They simply can't engage and are truly in hell. It's their baseline state and yet often they don't even realize that they're in it.

111

I never give up on anyone—ever! However, I don't know how to break through this firewall of anger on a consistent basis. I have been successful a few times but when I fail it's brutal. I have significant anxiety dealing with extremely angry patients and am trying to learn better strategies. I am open to suggestions.

CHAPTER 7

Reprogramming the Nervous System

All pain is "in your head." I don't mean that it's imaginary; it's just that every pain impulse has to be interpreted by your brain. Although your emotions do affect your perception of pain, you didn't imagine the sensation, and it's not "psychological." What happens with repetitive pain impulses is that your nervous system lays down pathways that become very efficient. Thus, your body becomes "programmed" to feel a certain way. My ultimate goal is to help you "reprogram" your nervous system to essentially undo those pain pathways

THE TALENT CODE

The Talent Code, by Dan Coyle, is a book that sheds light on the reprogramming process in a fascinating way.[1] I now recommend it to all my patients because the author links the laying down of neurologic pathways to recent research in neuroscience. He discusses how practicing certain skills in a certain way creates pathways that lead to deep learning. This deep learning is akin to the repetition of pain impulses and negative thoughts that you experience while in chronic pain. Just as a violinist in *The Talent Code* becomes skilled at playing the violin over hundreds of hours of practice, you can literally become "skilled" at experiencing pain and negativity. Conversely, you can also become skilled at laying down new, positive pathways through the reprogramming techniques that I'll cover in this chapter.

To better understand the concept of deep learning, consider a major league baseball player. The typical player can hit a ball that's coming at him between seventy and a hundred miles per hour, with varying trajectories. But only a small percentage of players can get a hit over 30% of the time. It takes tens of thousands of swings for that ability to become ingrained. Unfortunately, with chronic pain the number of "swings" it takes to gain the "skill" of memorizing that pain can probably be completed in just a few weeks.

The brain can create new connections at any age, an ability called neuroplasticity. One substance in the brain that contributes to the creation of these pathways is called myelin. Myelin is secreted in response to a stimulus and "etches in" the combination of neurons required to perform any task. Layers of myelin wrap around the pathways, not unlike insulation wraps around a wire, selectively improving the conductivity of those pathways. The thicker the insulation, the more efficient the pathway.

The Talent Code is extremely useful in changing your perception of how the brain works. My patients have found it helpful to learn how the nervous system possesses a mechanism that allows it to memorize thoughts and actions. This knowledge allows them to better conceptualize their pain and response to pain in terms of programmed pathways. Then, by using reprogramming tools, they can create "detours" around the old pathways, ones that do not include pain.

PROGRAMMING/REPROGRAMMING

To understand how programming works, first consider that it starts in the initial ten to twelve years of life, when our brains absorb everything in our environment. Negative behaviors and attitudes from our parents, friends, teachers, advertising, etc.

seep into our consciousness. We also adopt labels, some of them negative, for almost every component of our lives, including ourselves. As discussed earlier in the book, once the negative labels are there, they evolve to become our "stories." New and ongoing stimuli are interpreted through our labeling, which reinforces these stories.

You also have a story about your chronic pain. I would venture to guess that it's not a positive story. Most of these stories are, in fact, quite dark; the only variable I find is how well patients think they can hide their story from me and the pain psychologists with whom I collaborate.

Your story about chronic pain differs from your other stories in that it's associated with a physical sensation. This association makes the story particularly intense. The sensation of pain sparks negative thinking, which reminds you of your pain, which brings you back to your negative thoughts, and so on, creating a new neurological pathway that is reinforced with repetition. The more repetition, the better the brain becomes at processing these pathways; they will even adapt to resist being broken or derailed.

As we covered in earlier chapters, it's not helpful to cope with repetitive negative thoughts by suffering, suppressing them, or masking them with obsessive behavior. To really break the cycle, you have to reprogram your thoughts. In my experience with thousands of patients, it's the only method that works.

Our brains are complex computers that are programmable. To effectively take part in the reprogramming process, it's critical to understand that we can control it. First, you have to become familiar with all the programs that are already running in your brain. This involves breaking down the defenses that are keeping your story about chronic pain beneath the surface.

There are three phases to forming alternative neurological pathways: 1) increasing awareness of the thought or pattern of thoughts that incites your pain, 2) detaching from the thought, and 3) burning a pathway of new and different thoughts.

INCREASING AWARENESS OF PATTERNS OF THINKING

Becoming aware of your negative thoughts starts with identifying the actual stressor. This may seem obvious: "My son got his girlfriend pregnant. That's what's causing my stress." However, it's more complicated than that. By stressor, I'm referring to the specific aspect of the situation that's causing you to feel upset. Your son did not physically harm you or insult you. While he is your child, he *is* living his own life. And it shouldn't be a surprise that teenagers engage in sexual activity. It may directly affect you in that you'd feel obligated to provide physical and emotional support. It's your choice whether to do so, however.

So what's upsetting you? Perhaps it's that he violated your belief system; maybe you'd hammered away at him about the immorality of pre-marital sex and you're upset he didn't take your belief to heart; or he might've upset your image of the perfect family. For many cultures, however, this situation wouldn't be a problem. Some parents are actually excited to have a grandchild whether or not there has been a wedding. The bottom line is that you are working from your *own* frame of reference.

It isn't a matter of being right or wrong, but rather realizing that if you're feeling stressed about a situation, it's critical to step back and look at it more closely. Be clear on what part of the problem is the source of the stress.

The simplest way to increase awareness of why you're stressed is to describe in writing both the situation and exactly how it makes you feel. This is a powerful strategy. You can also use meditation, or talk to a counselor, confidant, etc. Doing so will allow you to separate your reaction from the event.

Remember, there's the situation that might be upsetting, there's your reaction, and there's you. By separating these components you can consider things more clearly so that the situation at hand doesn't escalate into a crisis.

Note that writing about anything that's occurred in your life has a tendency to cause anxiety, initially. By acknowledging your thoughts and feelings, you may be tapping into some deep-seated issues. However, they are actually not "issues." They are just more irrational circuits that you cannot change. That is one of the beauties of this process. There's nothing about yourself that you have to analyze and fix. As you engage in these strategies your nervous system will re-wire—and so heal—itself.

DETACHING FROM THE CIRCUIT

The following is a light story from my life that's an example of how you cannot change existing circuits. The only possibility is to detach and re-route.

> *I don't remember much about learning how to ride a bicycle; I only remember something about training wheels and taking a few nasty falls after they came off. I do know that my father wasn't there to help me or witness it. He was a small-town family doctor who routinely worked over a hundred hours a week.*
>
> *I think that I must be traumatized by not having my father around when I accomplished this rite of passage. In fact, the longer I sit here thinking about it, the more upset I think I am getting. What do you think I should do?*
>
> *One option would be to talk to someone about this childhood trauma. Do I have an unconscious stress response when I even just see a bicycle? Maybe that's why I never took up serious cycling. I don't know if I should talk to a psychologist about this experience or to a trainer to unlearn how to ride a bike. The latter would be more effective. I wonder how long it would take me to unlearn this skill. I am sure I would have a better life.*

Unfortunately, you can't unlearn how to ride a bicycle. It's impossible to eliminate the neurological pathways associated with the experience. In fact, you can't eliminate any of your past experiences from your brain. Most of your lifetime just sits there, and any part of it can be triggered by a word, comment, or image. The links to the part triggered in memory also cannot be broken.

Pain pathways are the same as the bicycle pathways. They can't be eliminated, and neither can the associated experiences. It's all bound tightly together. The continued assault of pain only makes the pathways more intractable.

What are you going to do?

The best way to move beyond stress, after becoming aware of it, is to detach from it. Actually, it's your only choice. A common coping strategy when we're stressed is to try and control our environment so we don't have to be exposed to the stressor any longer. It eventually becomes very stressful trying avoid stress, though. If you can detach and learn not to respond to negative thought patterns, they will eventually lose a lot of their power. They may not disappear, but they'll have much less control over you.

In addition to helping increase awareness, writing is also a powerful way to help you detach. With awareness, you write about what you're feeling (as above). To detach, write about the effect that the negative thought/feeling is having on your quality of life. For instance, you might see that if you remained angry with your son for getting his girlfriend pregnant, you'd run the risk of damaging your relationship with him and your future grandchild. This would help you decide to not remain in that initial frame of mind.

Detachment via meditation involves watching thoughts come in and out of your mind and learning not to respond to them. You observe the thoughts as a separate entity, without reacting.

A third way to detach is to envision a negative thought and connect it to an unpleasant physical sensation. This is a method that originated in the Hoffman Process. Associating thought patterns with a physical sensation creates an alternate neurologic pathway.

ETCHING NEW PATHWAYS

Awareness and detachment just begin the reprogramming process. The third step in reprogramming is to create circuits in your brain that are more functional and appropriate to a given situation. This is etching a new pathway. (I also call it "connected thinking.") For instance, a father of a teenage son with a pregnant girlfriend could etch a new pathway by saying, "This situation is challenging but I love my son. Whatever we decide, I will not let this negatively affect our relationship and family dynamic." The father does not have to like the situation or agree that it's being handled in the best way; he just has to be aware of his reactions and solve the problem based *only* on what it presents in and of itself. This process is much different than positive thinking, a common—and commonly unsuccessful—method employed to suppress negative thoughts.

Writing is the most effective method to start etching new pathways. With writing, you are associating thoughts with a physical sensation. Visualization is also effective but it's a more advanced skill.

I often use this metaphor with my patients: Picture your brain sitting on a table with billions of pathways etched into it, many of them very strong. Your life outlook and sense of well-being are contained in this mass of tissue that weighs just a few pounds. Imagine trying to suppress all of this brain activity. You can't cover it with a "blanket" of positive thinking and expect to change it in any life-altering way.

Now picture a second brain that's processing only your basic bodily functions. You can engrave new pathways into it that are more functional. Creating these new pathways takes repetition and commitment, though. This process is much more proactive than simply analyzing the old brain. As you create your new reality, the new brain will become more active and the old brain will begin to atrophy. Envision the new brain in twelve to eighteen months, when it is vibrant, creative, and in charge. With this new model, you will no longer have to fight with your old neurological pathways.

Brain Size

Speaking of brains, it's well documented that patients suffering from chronic pain experience a significant decrease in the size of their brains. It's unclear exactly why this occurs, but it's a consistent observation. It makes sense to me that if much of your brain is stuck in the repetitive thought patterns associated with pain, other parts—the ones that experience good friends, wine, food, experiences, etc.—will atrophy. It has also been shown that the phenomenon is reversible with active intervention such as reprogramming. Chronic pain sucks the life right out of you—including brain cells. Don't let that process continue![2]

THE TOOLS

Let's talk more about writing and awareness. I believe that these reprogramming methods can and should be more systematically utilized by mainstream medicine. Specifics about the application of these techniques will be described in upcoming chapters. Following are some general principles:

Writing

As established earlier in the book, we are not our thoughts. But although we may be able to grasp this concept intellectually, it's harder to accept it in the course of our day-to-day lives. In fact, the most formidable obstacle I face daily is trying to get patients to understand that their thoughts do not define them. The ones who do, move forward. The others remain stuck—really stuck.

To reiterate, one powerful way to disconnect from your thoughts is through writing. When you write down a thought, you're immediately creating a physical space between you and that thought. That *space* is then associated with the physical sensations of vision and touch. Somehow your nervous system can internalize that space, helping you detach from your swirling, racing thoughts. The opposite effect occurs when you attempt to accomplish this in your head.

Writing is the starting point of the whole DOCC program. NOTHING will occur in terms of reprogramming your thoughts on your path to good health until you begin to write. There are many additional tools but no substitutes.

The technique that almost single-handedly pulled me out of my personal crisis was the "three-column" method outlined in *Feeling Good* by David Burns.[3] I recommend Burns's writing exercises to all of my patients. I've noticed that patients who fully engage in writing see a decrease in their anxiety very quickly. They typically respond within two to four weeks.

The three-column technique represents the three phases of reprogramming: 1) awareness, 2) detachment, and 3) creation of a new pathway.

The three columns are:

Negative thought   *Error in thinking*   *Rational Thought*

By writing your negative thought in the first column, you are increasing your awareness of the problem.

An error in thinking could be any number of things, including "should thinking," "labeling," "mind reading," "catastrophizing," etc. Categorizing your error allows you to see what it's doing to your quality of life. This represents the detaching process. You then have a choice to either continue that line of thinking or to "re-structure" your thoughts. In the third column, the more rational follow-up thought is written down, creating a new neurologic pathway.

Here's an example of the three-column technique in action. Consider the fact that it's common for spouses to have different views on punctuality. You might always be on time while your spouse is habitually late. In this scenario, you'd likely have a similar set of thoughts every time he was late, such as, "My time isn't being respected" or "He's always late. He's a really inconsiderate person."

If your spouse was late to meet you for an event one night and you were still stewing about it afterward, here's one way to process the situation. Get out a piece of paper, create three columns, and then fill them in:

Negative thought	Error in thinking	Rational Thought
Inconsiderate	Labeling	I don't know why he was late. We'll discuss it later.

In addition to seeing your spouse as inconsiderate, you might have racing thoughts like, "This being late is really unacceptable," or "I'm really angry." These thoughts can spin for a long time. (And you can do the technique with them as well.) You may have the same or similar thoughts the next time the lateness occurs, but, by doing the writing repeatedly, their frequency and intensity will diminish. You can then solve the situation in a rational way separate from your initial reaction to it.

By writing about the situation, you are separating from your thoughts via touch and feel, and forming new pathways. I personally have yet to find a shortcut and have not yet seen a patient who could bypass this step and become pain-free.

Positive Thinking and Suppression

The lateness scenario above has many layers and can be considered from many different angles. Writing helps you process your lingering frustration, but how would you handle the situation in the moment? First, there's suppression. Suppose you're going out on a date later that evening; you have two hot tickets to a play that you've anticipated for months. If your spouse shows up late, you may be upset but, because you don't want to ruin the date, you might decide to just "stuff" your feelings of frustration, pretend he wasn't late, and proceed with the evening. The chances of really enjoying yourself at a deep level, however, have diminished. Even though you've suppressed your feelings, they are still there somewhere, simmering below the surface. They may not surface that night, but they will emerge in some form over the long term. Suppression is a bad idea all around.

Or you might try positive thinking, something along the lines of, "I really love my spouse. He has some faults but there are many more positives." This doesn't work either. Although these thoughts are rational and they might calm you somewhat, they're not an effective way to deal with the root problem. You cannot control your mind *with* your mind consistently over the long term, or, in other words, you can't "out-think" your own thoughts. If you're upset, you're upset. More importantly, see how much mental energy you can waste on just one situation.

In the next section on awareness, you'll learn about a method called "active meditation," which helps you to calm your mind with your body. It allows you to become an observer of your own reactions and begin to see yourself the way others see you. It's a tool you can use again and again in the midst of the chaos of your mind.

Awareness/Meditation

We will discuss meditation and awareness in detail in Chapter 8. Here I'll provide a brief overview so you can see how it fits into reprogramming.

Meditation is an effective reprogramming tool because the goal is to train your brain to be fully present in the moment. There are many different types of meditation and awareness; the key is to find the one to which you feel the strongest connection.

I, personally, practice active meditation, a technique where I consciously work on hearing, seeing, and feeling every aspect of whatever is in front of me. It has the dramatic effect of pulling my head out of my stories and connecting me to the present.

Another method is structured meditation, where you might concentrate on just breathing. When you focus solely on your breath, you are fully present in that moment. Invariably, outside negative thoughts will arise. As discussed previously, it's important to just "watch" the thought enter your mind and allow it to stay there for as long as it wants. In the meantime, you draw your attention back to your breathing. As the thought leaves, you'll return to the present moment.

The detachment process occurs as you watch the thoughts come and go. You learn to not be affected by the intensity or frequency of these thoughts and subsequent emotions.

It's easy to construe some of these practices as "positive thinking," but they are the opposite. With meditation, as you watch the sometimes disturbing thoughts enter your mind, you might often experience some deep emotional reactions. Over time, you become better at letting these thoughts and feelings go, but at the beginning it can be unsettling. In any case, you learn how to "fail" in meditation and still be okay with it. This is unlike positive thinking, where you'd try to suppress any troubling thoughts or emotions.

Meditation and awareness practices will add a very powerful dimension to your life and your mental health.

Visualization

When you're in chronic pain, visualization can help you see a new life for yourself. Part of the chronic pain experience is feeling stuck, like your life will never change. But if you can picture a different existence—a time when you can move with greater ease and do more things, you can change your world. Visualizing a different way of living is a way to detach from your feelings of anxiety and reprogram your brain to get closer to a more functional state.

Visualization techniques have been used in the athletic and performing arts worlds for many years and there have been numerous studies demonstrating the effectiveness of these methods.

My son, Nick, was on the US developmental ski team as a mogul skier. As I've mentioned, he's an excellent skier and has come close to making it all the way to the top. He and his best friend, Holt, have enhanced their performance skills by utilizing both awareness and visualization in training. By using these techniques, they have not only elevated their performances, but have improved their ability to handle the inevitable failures that are inherent in any sport.

In March of 2007, our family was watching the competition for the US national championship in moguls. Nick had had a bad day and did not make the finals. Everyone, including Holt, was pretty upset. Nick had been talked into trying a trick he hadn't mastered, and he just didn't make it. Holt had a great run and qualified second. The top skier on the US ski team had qualified third. The top twelve skiers out of a field of fifty get a second run. There is no carry-over of points from the first run.

It was around 4:00 in the afternoon by the time the final run was winding down. The sun was low and the light was flat. Flat light makes it much harder to see the shapes of the moguls. The top US skier took his run and it was almost flawless. He scored a 27.2 out of a possible score of 30. Usually a score above 26.5 has a high chance of being the winning score. Holt was the next skier. We all were wishing him the best but just hoped that he would have a good run and possibly finish second or third. He came out, scored a 27.6, and won the US championship. We were ecstatic and dumbfounded. It was an incredible run under any circumstances, but almost impossible to pull off under those conditions and that kind of pressure. At that point, I didn't really understand the visualization process and how it was different from positive thinking. So I spent the next day picking Holt's brain, asking how he was able to perform so well.

Here's what he told me. It is first of all critical for the performer to acknowledge the anxiety associated with the upcoming performance. Holt was very anxious and knew that the score he had to beat was high. However, instead of suppressing his anxiety he stuck with it and experienced it. He made a simple and quick choice: "I am not going to be controlled by any negative thoughts or emotions." He then turned his attention to active meditation. He felt the wind on his face and listened to the sound of his skis pushing against the snow. He felt himself breathe and just put himself onto the pathway he had visualized so many times. He didn't visualize himself on the winner's podium, but rather focused on being present during the actual run itself. The former is positive thinking and would have distracted him from executing at his best. He had been practicing these techniques the whole season.

In the past, Holt said, his strategy would have been to suppress his negative emotions with thoughts like, "Don't worry about the other skier's score," "Don't be nervous" or "I can do it." The energy spent on trying to deny and cover up his real feelings would've taken away from the energy and focus he needed to perform. He instead chose an alternate neurological pathway that was the one he needed to maximize his performance.

The reprogramming that Holt did through visualization is a powerful method that is a little more advanced than writing exercises: with visualization, you experience the entire event in your head. It's the only program that's playing. It's important to go over each detail, from beginning to end.

Holt's method is validated by sports performance literature which states that "internal" visualization is more effective than "external" visualization. With internal visualization, you actually *feel* as if you are performing the athletic feat, whereas with external visualization, you are merely watching yourself perform the event. You should be trying to feel the air, hear the crowd, and feel as much of your body moving as possible, etc. The more senses you can experience in your mind, the better.

Visualization techniques can be applied to your life, not only in helping with your chronic pain but also in mundane day-to-day tasks.

THE DIFFERENCE BETWEEN
REPROGRAMMING AND PSYCHOLOGY

Twenty-five years ago, when I was living with severe OCD and chronic pain, I began to think that chronic pain was a type of obsessive disorder. Today I am convinced that this is the case. My basic definition of an obsessive disorder is unresolved anxiety fueled by anger.

OCD and other related disorders are considered incurable in the traditional psychiatric world. The focus is on treating the symptoms, without a lot of benefit. However I am a witness that OCD is curable. Chronic pain is curable.

Mainstream psychology and psychiatry are currently the most common ways to deal with mental health issues, including OCD and problems associated with chronic pain. The implication has been that your pain doesn't really exist; you're merely imagining it. There's also a tendency for others to think that you, the sufferer, are weak and/or have a "low pain threshold."

These assumptions are unfounded, however. In truth, the sensation of chronic pain is not a psychological problem. As discussed earlier, when you experience pain, the pain-related areas of your brain are firing away at a super-charged level. Again, the pain is NOT imaginary. Rather, your brain has been programmed to send pain signals to your nervous system. With repetition the brain will lay down pathways and become increasingly skilled in utilizing them.

Discussing pain-related issues in counseling can be helpful as an adjunct to using reprogramming tools, but it's not effective as a primary treatment. Talk therapy does not create new neurological pathways. In fact, talking brings the existing destructive pathways more to your attention and makes them more complex.

I believe that we should undergo a major paradigm shift in conceptualizing mental health. Addressing the mind-body connection through one of the many reprogramming strategies makes chronic pain curable. We can't predict when the symptoms will disappear, but when it occurs, it happens quickly and often radically.

MIND BODY SYNDROME

As discussed in Chapter 1, up until recently I'd heard about the Mind Body Syndrome for two decades but had never placed much credence in it. It didn't seem to fit any conceptual model of disease that I'd learned. I knew that stress could increase your chances of illness and severe disease, but I'd just assumed that the root problem of disease was a chronic imbalance of the body's chemistry caused by hormones released under stress. Now I see, however, that your brain also has the capacity to directly cause symptoms, including chronic pain. This happens because your nervous system is connected to every cell in the body by nerves or chemicals.

The basic premise of MBS is that a pain pathway is created within a unique set of circumstances. If a similar situation is re-encountered then the pain pathways can be re-stimulated, causing the exact set of symptoms to re-occur, usually with the same intensity.

In the book *Unlearn Your Pain*, Howard Schubiner tells the story of a physician who was injured while serving in the Vietnam War.[5] His helicopter was shot down and his left leg was crushed. Several surgeries later, he had an almost normally functioning leg. Once or twice a year, however, his leg would develop severe pain and swelling, lasting several days and sometimes up to a week. During these periods, he was quite incapacitated, but afterward his leg would return to normal. Every test for a new injury would come out negative.

One day he was walking with his wife in a park when the symptoms suddenly returned and he almost fell to the ground. His wife looked at him and asked, "Did you hear the helicopter?" He replied, no, he hadn't. His brain, however, *had*.

While this man's situation might seem like a psychological issue, it's not. He wasn't imagining his symptoms. Rather, the symptoms were linked to pain pathways that were triggered by his brain and nervous system. His initial injury had occurred while helicopters were flying overhead in Vietnam (the unique set of circumstances). When he met with similar circumstances, even if he did not consciously recognize them, the memory/pain pathways were re-stimulated.

There is another situation that can elicit symptoms. Remember that pain is always associated with anxiety and frustration. So instead of a specific circumstance causing a pain pathway to flare up, symptoms can be reignited by an increased level of anger or anxiety. Again, it's a linkage mechanism at work.

Schubiner provides a test in *Unlearn Your Pain* that allows you to determine if you have symptoms of the Mind Body Syndrome. Chronic pain is one possibility. Some of the others are:

- TMJ
- Migraine Headaches
- Irritable Bowel Syndrome
- Spastic bladder
- Tinnitus
- Fibromyalgia
- Reflux
- Obsessive thinking patterns
- Anxiety
- Unexplained rashes
- Burning sensations

I frequently see patients who've had a successful surgery but later suddenly return to my office with a recurrence of the same symptoms they experienced pre-surgery. I occasionally repeat the diagnostic testing, but most of the time I don't find a cause for the flare-up. Now I wait a few weeks to order the tests to see if some circumstance or particular stress has stimulated the old pain pathway. Often that's the case. Usually re-implementing the reprogramming tools will calm down the pain within a couple of days.

Pavlov's Dog

One experiment that demonstrates the power of reprogramming is the famous one by Ivan Pavlov, a Russian researcher.

Pavlov showed how the brain can be trained, through repetition, to have certain reactions in certain circumstances. His results further support the theories behind Mind Body Syndrome.

Pavlov set up a situation where every interaction a dog had with food would involve the sound of a bell. Eventually just the bell sound would cause the dog to salivate, even without seeing or smelling food.

One of Pavlov's lesser-known experiments is when he coupled the dog's interaction with food with an electric shock to one leg. With repetition, the dog would eventually seek the electric shock to obtain food and wouldn't react to the shock with a pain response. This phenomenon was "paw dependent" in that if the same shock was applied to its other leg, the dog would scream with pain.[6]

Why Is Reprogramming Your Only Option?

Once you have a pathway in your brain it will never disappear. It's similar to learning how to ride a bicycle: as per above, you cannot unlearn how to ride one. Pathways *will* atrophy with disuse, however. That's why it's so critical to understand the concept of reprogramming.

Fortunately, when it comes to pain the brain is hierarchal. It can only really focus on one thing at a time. There are some people who are remarkable in their ability to multi-task, but they can still only process a few things at once.

Consider that when you are driving home from work, your brain doesn't remember every car, house, and tree that you have passed. You might remember a yellow Ferrari or a major accident—these things catch your attention and move to the top of the hierarchy. But that's about it. Your brain is seeing all of it and screening out most of it.

The reprogramming tools in this book create a massive "shift" in your brain, to the point where your thoughts about living a full life are higher in the hierarchy. That's the whole point of the exercise. You want to get to a point where your brain is screening out everything except for a productive existence and there's little use for the old circuits that are connected to the pain pathways. The more fully engaged you are with incorporating these tools into your life on a long-term basis, the more effective the process.

In the reprogramming process, there are five stages of five steps each (as you'll see in Chapter 9). It appears that many patients experience a significant decrease in pain while working through Stage II, which is dealing with their anger. Anger seems to have a particularly strong link to chronic pain. This can create a problem, however, in that people tend to feel so much better at Stage II that they essentially quit the rest of the journey. It's vital to move through the whole process to create a shift in your brain for good.

I once witnessed the importance of full engagement in the case of one of my favorite patients, Vic. About ten years ago, Vic, at age thirty, experienced a ruptured disc and pinched nerve at the lowest level of his spine. He was urgently admitted to the hospital and underwent a fusion.

Vic was a finish carpenter, a job which involves lifting in difficult positions. Post-surgery, his leg pain continued to be quite severe but he was able to function reasonably well with low-dose narcotics. He also actively engaged in the writing process and worked with a pain psychologist. He was enthusiastic about developing stress management skills, which not only helped him cope with the pain, but also decreased it.

About nine months after his surgery, Vic was scheduled to start retraining for a new career. Then, six weeks before he started the program, his pain returned dramatically, to the point that I ordered an MRI of his back. The results showed no change from before. I sat down with him and he admitted that he'd stopped writing and was experiencing extreme anxiety about his ability to fully participate in the job retraining.

After our talk, he re-engaged with the writing and the pain psychologist. The pain rapidly decreased to his baseline level. It was interesting to both of us that once he started the job retraining program, his pain dropped down even more. His mind had been redirected to healthier and more interesting pathways.

Everyone wants to thrive—there is no exception. The only questions are how deeply is the "real you" buried and do you have the tools and motivation to reconnect with the person who *is* you.

By engaging in the reprogramming process, your anxiety/anger/pain will no longer be running your life. You can employ the tools on an ongoing basis, as needed, to remain in charge of your wellness and maintain your ability to live your life fully.

CHAPTER 8

Awareness

By now we've established that anxiety and anger are major aspects of the chronic pain experience, but awareness of your surroundings is another element we've yet to explore: Anxiety and anger cloud your awareness of what's going on around you and limit your ability to interact with others. When you are in that state, your mind is full of racing thoughts and vivid imagery and it's hard to focus on anything but your pain. This can make it a challenge for friends, family, and coworkers —anyone —to connect with you. If you're touchy and constantly on edge, it's exhausting for others to be in your presence. Having a good support system is an important part of your recovery from chronic pain because positive relationships have a calming effect. That's why it's critical to become more aware of your thoughts, emotions, words, actions, and reactions. What you're not aware of can and will control you. Understanding how anxiety and anger narrow your awareness and affect your relationships will help you to keep those external channels open. You can't eliminate anxiety and anger completely, but awareness will help you prevent them from running your life.

MEDITATION

Meditation strengthens awareness. In meditation, you use various methods to connect fully with the present moment. There are a multitude of techniques and schools of thought; one technique is to focus only on your breath, becoming aware of as many aspects of your breathing as you can. As you do this you'll become immersed in the moment. Various thoughts will enter your mind, but instead of being distracted, you simply watch them come and then watch them leave. The goal is to not to ignore these thoughts, but to learn not to react to them. This is the process of detachment. After the momentary distraction, you gently pull yourself back to your breathing as quickly as possible.

When you meditate, you don't slow down or control your racing thoughts. Instead, you "de-energize" them so that they have less control over you. As you develop the ability to stay in the present moment, the thoughts become less relevant and decrease—often dramatically. The key is to not try and edit, fix, or control them; that will only make them stronger.

LEVELS OF AWARENESS

Skilled masters have developed a profound depth of knowledge of meditation and awareness over thousands of years. I am just sharing some concepts and tools that I've found useful in the context of a life that is far too busy. I think of awareness from these four different perspectives:

- Environmental
- Emotional
- Storytelling/Judgmental
- Ingrained patterns

Each of these levels of awareness has been presented and discussed in almost every forum that deals with personal growth. I'm hopeful that you'll be motivated to pursue your own journey of awareness with an experienced teacher.

Environmental Awareness

Environmental awareness is using meditation to be fully aware of as many of your senses as possible as you go about your day. Or you can focus on just one of the senses. I call this active meditation, and it's obviously different from the most well-known types of meditation practice, where you typically go someplace peaceful and quiet. I've found that engaging in environmental awareness makes me more attuned to each of the three other types of awareness.

Being aware of your senses grounds you in your environment and has a calming effect on your nervous system. It also makes you more sensitive to different emotions that you're feeling. If you're not plugged into your own environment, you can be pushed around by your emotions and not realize how they're negatively affecting your day. Like most surgeons, I find it hard to sit still; active meditation has enabled me to be a calmer person and more effective in my job.

As a veteran spine surgeon with many years of experience, I'm referred many complicated spine problems that require complex surgeries. Like all surgeons, I have intermittent complications among my patients. Although I've been committed to having no complications from the first day I walked into the OR, there was a point a few years ago when I faced up to the fact that I hadn't been able to eliminate them entirely. This led me to develop a somewhat defensive mindset. If I could get through the week without a complication it was a huge relief. I was enjoying my time in the OR less and less.

Things changed when I decided to enlist the help of a performance coach, David Elaimy, to help me reduce any mistakes in surgery. This was a major turning point in my professional life. I brought David into the operating room and into the clinic to better understand my world, and for eighteen months he and I underwent regular debriefings and coaching. With David's help, I began to use active meditation in the OR.

David's basic model is that performance equals skill minus interference. My most common interferences in the OR were frustration, anxiety, distraction, complacency, and, especially, being in a rush to finish. They all detracted from the consistency of my performance. This model is based not on suppressing interference —for instance, if you're frustrated, you don't pretend otherwise —rather, you face these frustrations and then detach. Using tools and approaches that have been employed for centuries in the practices of meditation and mindfulness, I'm now able to identify any interference either before or during surgery, and then let go of it.

This is how it works: Each surgical morning, I wake up and assess how I'm feeling. Just as with everyone, it ranges from calm and relaxed to tired and anxious. Then I immediately start paying attention to every smell, touch, and taste possible. I feel the water on my back in the shower; I smell the coffee. I also remind myself that although today's surgery is "just another case" for me, it's one of the most important days of my patient's life. I continue the awareness process for a couple of hours, on into the OR. I carefully arrange the room and talk to each member of the surgical team. We re-review the imaging studies. Previously, I'd rush into the OR at the last minute just before making the incision. Now, by the time I start my case I'm usually focused and immersed in what's right in front of me.

During surgery, awareness is what allows me to perform each next move at an optimum level. I feel the pressure of my grip on each surgical tool; I notice the shape of the contours of the anatomy; I feel my shoulder and arm muscles and keep them relaxed; and I watch the flow of the case. If I feel any disruptive emotions intrude into my state of mind, I quickly practice my environmental awareness techniques in order to re-focus. I have learned to be more fully engaged on a higher percent of cases; I can "program" myself into "the zone."

Since I start practicing active meditation, my complication rate in surgery has noticeably decreased. For instance, from 1999 until 2003 I had an "acceptable" 9% rate (per year) of inadvertently entering the dural sac (a sack of fluid surrounding the brain and spinal cord in the skull and spinal column). In the last couple of years I've made this mistake only two or three times a year, which is about less than one percent.

Surgery has again become a wonderful experience for me. Now I eagerly look forward to Monday instead of Friday. I'm also more committed to getting a good night's sleep before my OR days. If I wake up "wired" and uneasy, I slow down until I feel relaxed (a relative word for a surgeon), no matter how many things are on my to-do list.

Through working with David I have changed my paradigm of spine surgery; the actual surgery feels more like creating a work of art. I am sculpting away the abnormal anatomy to create normal anatomy. Also, my staff is more relaxed. If a complication occurs, I know exactly what state of mind I'm in and can take full responsibility for it.

David and I have developed a seminar called "Awake at the Wound," in which we teach physicians and staff these performance principles. Many non-physicians have attended, since, in reality, performing in the OR is just one tightly compacted metaphor for managing life's stresses.

I also practice active meditation outside of the OR on a daily basis. Environmental awareness is more difficult in the less controlled areas of my life, but it is still my "go-to" practice of awareness.

One tool I use to practice awareness is my "to do" list. I remind myself that this list is an expression of my life, and so I practice being aware as I go about each item. For instance, when I have an appointment with a patient, I listen to myself talk to him or her. I feel the pen on the paper as I jot down notes. I also practice meditative techniques such as watching the intrusive thoughts of "need to finish up here, I have other things to do" enter my consciousness, and then leave. I remember that my goal is to engage and enjoy every second of my "to do" list. It doesn't always work, but it's surprising how often it does.

Environmental awareness engages me in the present moment regardless of the circumstances. My wish is to simply live my life at this level.

The Hurricane

One evening I came up with a metaphor that helped me better relate to my life stresses and remain in a peaceful state of mind. I call it "the eye of the hurricane."

I was watching the news about the progress of Hurricane Gustav as it approached New Orleans and the other Gulf States. In a hurricane, the winds are strongest at the periphery, but the eye is quiet. As I watched the satellite and radar pictures I realized that the whirling wind represented my repetitive racing thoughts. The further I get from the peaceful center, the larger impact these thoughts have on the quality of my day.

My historic coping mechanism would be to try to slow down or ignore the thoughts. That took a lot of energy, though, and most of the time I was unsuccessful. As I ran out of energy, the thoughts would race more. But if I become aware of my senses through active meditation, I can pull myself back into the present moment—i.e., the peaceful center of the storm—and watch the thoughts race. If I don't identify with the thoughts, keeping them separate from me, I have much more energy to experience and enjoy my day.

The same metaphor works for any situation that you may encounter. Most of our lives have circumstances whirling around us that we cannot control, yet we spend a lot of time and energy trying to control them. It takes a lot of effort to try to stop a hurricane; you're not going to win. If you can pull yourself into the center and just deal with one issue at a time, you'll tap into more internal strength. By becoming more fully aware and centered, you can be at peace.

Emotional Awareness

In the presence of chronic pain, connecting with your emotions is particularly critical. If your emotions are out of control, they will inflame your pain. Ideally, we'd all be aware of our emotional state at any given moment, but there are several obstacles in the way. First, we don't start from a neutral position, but rather live in our own frame of reference. If, for instance, you were raised in an anxiety-ridden, abusive household, anxiety would be your normal emotional state in adulthood. Until your anxiety spun completely out of control, it would be hard for you to be aware of how much it was driving your "normal" behavior. Second, none of us likes to experience negative emotions, so we tend to automatically deny or suppress them rather than come to terms with them. We find distractions to avoid connecting with reality.

It takes courage to identify your negative emotions. This is particularly true if you're feeling like a victim. "Victim" has a lot of negative connotations. Yet it's a universal part of the human condition.

In my experience, unless you actively choose a journey of self-discovery, you can't connect with your true emotional state. You can't see who you really are unless you commit to stepping outside of your mind and looking at yourself from a different perspective. Ask yourself these questions: "Am I open?" "Am I coachable?" "Can I really listen and feel?" This is a starting point. Beyond that, active meditation is remarkably effective for self-discovery, as are the writing exercises I advocate in this book. Then there's external help —it's impossible to evolve without it. There are self-help books, counseling, meditation, seminars, retreats, etc. Once you get in touch with what's going on in your mind, you can go on a very powerful journey.

Many, if not most, people choose not to take this journey. But they make this choice at their own peril: unfortunately, what you're not aware of will run your life. The result may well be a lot of suffering for the individual and those close to him or her.

Why don't more people pursue a path of self-discovery? It may be because in our culture, most of us spend a lot of emotional energy trying to look good to people around us. We also try to look good to ourselves. Truly connecting with your emotions is an act of humility; most people just don't want to do something so difficult and unpleasant. However, it's also extremely rewarding, and it makes life so much easier in the end. It helped me to recover from my own chronic pain.

Judgment/Storytelling

A third level of awareness revolves around judgment and storytelling, which can ramp up your emotions in any given situation. On this level, you create a "story" or a judgment about yourself, another person, or a situation. These judgments tend to be criticisms that are rough and inflexible.

The brain has a bad habit of focusing on negative judgments. We can categorize them into the ten "errors in thinking" outlined by David Burns in his book *Feeling Good*.[1] When we make these errors, we create stories out of circumstances that are often non-events. Burns calls these negative thoughts "ANTS," which stands for "automatic negative thoughts."

For example, imagine someone at work walked by you and didn't acknowledge you. You might think they're upset with you about a situation that occurred the day before. The error in thinking in this case would be "mind reading." You can't read other people's minds—it's possible that the person had just received some bad news and wasn't engaging with anyone. But you don't really know. If you make assumptions, you're wasting a lot of emotional energy.

Then there is the error of "labeling." For example, a frequently late spouse becomes "inconsiderate." A forgetful teenager becomes "irresponsible." In the act of labeling, especially negative labeling, you're overlooking circumstances and others' good qualities, limiting your capacity to enjoy being with them.

Then there are the labels we have for ourselves: you knock something over and call yourself "clumsy." In addition to labeling, this error falls under "should" thinking. If a lover breaks up with you, then you're "unlovable." Rehashing these critical judgments in our minds turns them into deeply embedded stories.

Such stories are much harder to move on from than single judgments. Once a judgment sets into a story, you tend to lose all perspective. Over time, faulty thinking can become your reality.

In my own experience, whenever I have an "ANT," I become either angry or anxious (or both). I am also sometimes more reactive or impulsive. These emotions then fuel the thought and it becomes repetitive. As the thought keeps whirling around, it becomes stronger, along with my emotions. The resultant intensity can quickly destroy my day and negatively affect my relationships.

I've heard this thought pattern described as a "vicious cycle," a "whirlpool," etc. These kinds of thoughts, or stories, can become recurrent and might last for years. They take on a life of their own even though they are often fairly outrageous.

Regardless of what sets these patterns of thinking off, they are a universal part of the human experience. This is true whether chronic pain is involved or not. With chronic pain you have the added frustration of the physical stimulus to keep these circuits really spinning.

To better understand the story concept, consider common situations where the brain focuses on a self-perceived flaw that is not physically painful. It might be your height, weight, the shape of your body, or even an individual body part. Or it might be some particular quality, such as a lack of intelligence, athletic skill, musical talent, etc. Thinking about it over and over snares you in a destructive cycle of spinning neural circuits. For example, many years ago I had a patient with neck pain who was absolutely convinced that he was "stupid." His self-labeling wasn't rational, as he was clearly a bright guy. I don't know if his view of himself somehow triggered it, but he eventually developed a significant chronic burning sensation around his mouth.

Something similar often happens in the entertainment industry, where performers commonly focus only on their negative reviews. My wife, who is a tap dancer, has seen this in her profession for years. She pointed out to me that a performer might have ninety-nine positive reviews but will fixate on the one that's negative. In fact, it's a common saying that "you're only as good as your worst critic."

Another common, perhaps universal, phenomenon is focusing on a spouse's or partner's negative trait or traits. The other person usually has innumerable positive qualities that are forgotten in the face of the flaw. Over time the "story" can become so strong it can break apart an otherwise great relationship.

What's curious to me is why the human brain does not become equally fixated on positive traits. Reconsidering Wegner's "white bears" experiment, maybe it's because we don't suppress positive thoughts. As proven in his experiment, fixation goes hand in hand with suppression.

When I think of judgment and storytelling, one particular event from my own life comes to mind. It shows how creating stories has the power to disrupt your peace of mind and detract from your enjoyment of life.

One day my wife and I were taking my father for a ride up to beautiful Point Reyes, located on the coast north of San Francisco. About twenty minutes into our trip I noticed that the car's low-tire-pressure light had come on. It was a brand new car with only a thousand miles on it, so I thought it was probably just a malfunctioning light. I wasn't convinced that we'd made the correct decision to buy this car in the first place—it was more expensive than I was comfortable with—so I was more than a little frustrated that the light had a glitch.

I did stop to put a little air in the tire, just in case, and then kept driving for another forty-five minutes. As we approached Point Reyes in the early afternoon, however, we realized that the tire was really low, so I pulled over to change it. But when I opened the trunk, there was no spare. The story in my head was starting to ramp up as I wondered in frustration why a new car wouldn't have a spare. I called the car company's roadside assist line and they told me these new cars had "run-flat" tires that should be good for 150 miles at a maximum of fifty miles per hour. I felt a little insecure about that concept. We were a long way from the last large town we'd passed, and I thought that we should turn back. My wife thought that since my father rarely made it out from the East, we should go out to dinner. So we headed toward a restaurant on the coast. About three miles down the road the tire exploded.

It was now about four o'clock in the afternoon and we were miles and miles from anywhere. Our only option was to get towed back courtesy of AAA. It was hard for me to process the fact that I had to get my new car towed for a flat tire. The tow truck driver showed up to take us to the service station and let the three of us ride in the cab with my wife sitting on my lap. She started to complain about the bumpiness of the ride, which I found a little annoying. "I'm the one on the bottom," I thought. She wanted to have dinner in San Rafael and take a taxi home. I started to grind my teeth to keep my mouth shut.

This is how the afternoon had unfolded for me. Starting with the low tire, I'd made a decision to enjoy my time with my family in spite of the problem. I took note of my frustrations and concentrated on listening to the conversation and staying involved in the day. I was successful for a while—until the tire blew up. Then my anger began to bubble. I became aware that in spite of everything I'd learned about dealing with stress, I was greatly magnifying the problem with the thoughts in my head. I was thinking things like ,"I can't believe I got talked into buying this car," "My wife made me buy it," "It's me at the bottom of this pile; why are *you* the one complaining?" and "The tow truck driver must think we're out of our minds."

Although there might've been *some* truth in the things I was telling myself, I recognized that it wasn't helping us get through the situation. Nonetheless, I wasn't able to minimize my suffering through the stress relief techniques that had helped in the past, which was frustrating. I tried to talk myself out of it: "I know better. I can't control any of these variables right now, so let it go. I know how to do this." But it didn't work.

Then I began to go really dark with thoughts like, "How can I be married to this woman?" I began to notice how irrational and big these thoughts had become. It felt like a bomb had exploded. I was miserable way out of proportion to the situation.

In this incident, I was guilty of multiple errors in thinking. They came in the form of labeling, for instance—"My wife is irresponsible"—and catastrophizing—"Why did we get married?" Through it all, I negated her many positive qualities. To cite one, she's great at keeping things light, no matter what the problem, and unlike me, she was able to keep her cool throughout the day.

Historically I would've remained in this agitated state of mind for days with some carryover lasting for weeks. I wouldn't have been able to separate my wife's actions from my thoughts and realize that the problem wasn't her, it was my reaction to the situation. It was a major step for me to become aware of how out of proportion the story in my head had become. This degree of awareness really changed the game for me.

Eventually, we did get towed home. We went out to dinner. I still love my wife.

I learned yet another lesson in humility.

Ingrained Patterns

The behaviors we develop over a lifetime of exposure to our environment are what I call ingrained patterns. They stem from our upbringing and the fact that our brain is somewhat "hard-wired" during our formative years. For any given person, certain situations will elicit a fairly predictable response.

Our family interactions in childhood are at the root of how we act as adults. Certain situations in a given person's life will elicit a fairly predictable response based on that person's upbringing. We are hard-wired enough that we don't recognize or "feel" these patterns; it's just what we do. It's behavior that sits under many layers of defenses and has to be "dug out" by each person. I think our family-influenced habits and actions are much more obvious to our spouses and immediate family than they are to us; we can only get in touch with them through counseling, seminars, psychotherapy, self-reflection, spousal feedback, etc. Again, what you are not aware of will control you. Recognizing your own overall patterns is important.

Here is one example from the performance arena (at my work). (My wife could give you dozens in the personal arena.) A few years ago in the operating room I became aware that I consistently started to speed up towards the end of each case. I also realized that over the years, probably 80% of my dural tears had occurred in the last thirty minutes of a long case. The fatigue factor needs to be taken into account, but I think the speed issue is more critical. I still often don't notice that I speed up; I need feedback from my partners or assistants, so I ask them to act as my coaches. I'll stop for a few seconds and say, "Okay, the difficult part's done. It would be easy for me to relax and speed up to finish. Please speak up if you see me starting to rush." Every move in spine surgery is critical, so I have to make the choice to slow down. The end of a case is just as important as the beginning and middle.

This is just a brief overview of how, in my view, awareness plays a role in everyday life. It's something of a paradox in that when one is truly immersed in the moment there are no levels of awareness. It's just complete engagement-in-the-present-moment awareness. Maybe the concept should be called levels of "non-awareness." There's much more that can be discussed; I hope this is a starting point in your exploration of these ideas.

Becoming Aware of Your "Unawareness"

When I look back on my life's journey, one of the most disturbing aspects of doing so is realizing the extent of my *un*awareness. For instance, when I was in my full-blown obsessive mode, I didn't have a clue. I recall one time when a friend referred to my "obsessive nature." I didn't know what the word really meant, but whatever sense I had of it, I was certain it didn't apply to me.

How can you tap into your unawareness? One way is to look for cues in certain behaviors and attitudes that may mean you're out of touch with how you're feeling. Some examples:

- Having a rigid opinion about almost anything: religion, politics, someone's character, etc.
- Being told you're stubborn or "not listening"
- Interrupting someone to offer an opinion before you've heard theirs in total
- Insisting on being right
- Thinking about something besides what you're doing
- Judging yourself or others negatively or positively
- Feeling anxious or angry (once these feelings have been recognized and acknowledged in your life)
- Giving unasked-for advice
- Thinking you're wiser than your children
- Acting on impulse

This list goes on and on. If you notice more than one of these, it's probably time to take a step back and connect to your emotions so that you can respond appropriately to a given person or situation. This is the essence of awareness.

One of these cues, self-judgment, was a big part of my life and a major sign that I was unaware of my own patterns. It happened during my period of severe burnout, which lasted for several years. During that era, I had endless self-doubts and negative judgments about almost every aspect of my life. A severe case of perfectionism didn't help the situation. I often thought how much better it would be if I could judge myself positively with as much fervor.

I did change my life around. I learned a lot and have been able to help many people by drawing on the lessons I learned in barely surviving a severe depression. My practice has grown and I have an excellent reputation. I really enjoy my family and friends. It's great to enjoy the fruits of one's labors. However, as soon as I go into a mode of "what a compassionate guy I am" or "what a great surgeon I am" it takes me right down. Any effort on my part to spin my life in a positive way to others drains me of the energy I need to be creative and also distracts me from being aware of what's occurring right in front of me. For me, it turns out that positive self-judgment is just as disruptive as negative self-judgment. It's still judgment. What's truly enjoyable for me is to just be fully present for my next experience.

Another cue of unawareness, not listening, is one that I discovered with others' help. My weakness in this area became readily apparent one time when I attended a parents' meeting for my daughter's school, Hyde. I will preface this story by saying that I had always considered myself a good listener—it was one of my major personal identities. My wife, historically, has not agreed with that viewpoint. Of course I didn't listen to her.

At the meeting, we did one exercise where we had to write down on a piece of paper a characteristic that another parent "could work on." We could write to two parents and did not include our names. (This is one of those types of "games" that you are not anxious to win.) Most parents received one or two slips of paper. I received twelve (out of eighteen) that all said the same thing: "David, you don't know how to listen."

That was a very difficult moment for me. I found it extremely hard to not become defensive, but on the other hand, how could I disagree with twelve people? I came to accept that they were right, especially in retrospect. It was a trait that I truly could not see. I simply had to trust a group of people who I knew did not have an agenda and had my best interests at heart. After that meeting, I came to realize how not listening had interfered with my general awareness. It's one of the central tenets of awareness: *You cannot be aware if you cannot listen.*

The definition of awareness that resonates most with me is "being fully present in the moment." In other words, I'm most aware when I'm able to listen, feel, and observe multiple cues and then appropriately respond to the person or situation.

Unawareness and the Essence of Abuse

I discussed the link between pain, anger, and abuse in Chapter 6 and would like to re-emphasize the connection in this chapter. Abuse has a lot to do with awareness. Very few people who abuse others do it intentionally. They are usually consumed with anxiety-driven anger and are simply unaware of anyone else's needs. Their needs supersede all others' needs.

I had a patient many years ago who assaulted his grandmother for money. He was addicted to narcotics and needed the money to obtain drugs. When he was in my office he was personable and usually pretty rational. The difficulties started when I began to wean him off of his narcotics. He eventually threatened to kill me when I refused to give him medications at the level he wanted. We had to call the police and put our clinic under guard. His addiction had enveloped him to the point where he could only see his own needs.

I only became aware of how strongly chronic pain is connected to abuse after I had a long conversation with my father about my mother's abusiveness. Even though I saw medications all over the house growing up, I hadn't comprehended that she was in chronic pain. Between her rages she was an incredibly committed mother and she did have a lot of remorse after each and every episode of her abusive behavior. I am now very aware of the link and I'm direct with my patients about this problem.

The major obstacle to breaking through a given patient's unawareness of their own abusive behavior is that they simply don't recognize their anger and don't see their actions towards those close to them as abusive. They think that they're just expressing their legitimate frustrations. Becoming aware that your behavior might be considered abusive is tough. It's not how you'd like others to perceive you, and certainly not how you'd like to perceive yourself. No one would like it to be part of their self-image. Yet this awareness is absolutely critical.

Often people who are abusive "make up" for it by being pillars of the community or a church. They may hold an elevated position. Maybe they are very active in a charity. One of the worst sexual abuse cases I dealt with was perpetrated by a man who was a teacher, an elder in his church, and very vocal about how others should live their lives. Remember that one of the disguises of anger is "being right" or "living life with conviction." Eventually it came to light that he had been actively sleeping with his daughter from when she was five until she was fifteen. When it was all revealed, about twenty years later, his remorse was extreme. In his mind he had been a very committed father.

Verbal abuse is extremely common but recognized by few. It can be just as devastating as any other type of abuse, though. Being critical on a regular basis is the essence of it, but it's inherent in other behaviors as well: withholding words of affection, being silent, or not saying anything to actively help family members enjoy their day are also common, and more subtle, forms of verbal abuse. Also, any time you blame someone for creating your unhappiness and let them know it, you're probably being verbally abusive. You are the only one responsible for your happiness—end of story. The problem is very clearly outlined in a book, *Verbal Abuse—Survivors Speak Out,* by Patricia Evans.[2]

To have healthy and happy relationships, it's vital to work on being aware of others' needs every day.

Putting the Awareness Model to Work

We all want to become better, happier people and work pretty hard at it. As discussed, the marketing world keeps reminding us that we haven't met our potential and holds up endless images of perfection to reinforce that idea. We're led to believe that we need a better appearance, more friends, a longer list of accomplishments, more public recognition, greater power, etc. The message is "if I had more (or less) of 'X' I would be a happier person." (The list includes "less pain.") We are programmed into being defined by external factors.

Additionally, pressure from self-help resources is everywhere. Many of these resources claim to have all the answers. I fully support the use of external resources to help you on your journey to self-awareness, but it's important not to imagine that a single one of them is the remedy for all your problems. Of course, I offer many self-help tools in this book. But that's one of the paradoxes of this project. Even though I present methods for decreasing your pain and enhancing wellness, it's important to approach these methods with the right mindset. Truth is, the harder you try to "fix" yourself, the less likely you are to be successful in becoming pain-free. It's better to focus on enjoying your day with the idea that your pain or your life circumstances may *never* improve. In other words, you must learn to enjoy life with what you have right now.

If you're waiting for more wisdom, more reprogramming tools, more money, a nicer spouse, better-behaved kids, or less pain *before* you can fully engage in your life, it's never going to happen. It's illogical to think that all the variables in our lives will align so well that we'll have perfect fulfillment. And even if it *could* happen, how long do you think it would last? Think how much energy we spend trying to control so much.

You'll boost your energy if you focus on enjoying your day in spite of your current life circumstances. This extra energy leads to creativity, which helps you build the life you desire. I routinely do this exercise with my patients: I look at my watch and point out that the time is "X" and they have "Y" number of hours left in the day, then I ask them to make a decision to enjoy the next number of hours regardless of their circumstances.

How do you enjoy your day? A few simple suggestions: be kind and patient with others; be kind and patient with yourself; keep things in perspective, no matter what annoyances you encounter; take time to appreciate any good things that come your way, such as a warm greeting from a partner/friend or a good meal. There are many other examples, but you get the idea.

When I was in the middle of my own intense burnout about ten years ago I had to make a conscious decision, over and over, just to enjoy the next fifteen minutes. I'm not kidding. After all, I had to start somewhere. Gradually, though, I worked my way up to enjoying a full day.

My challenge to myself and to all of my patients is, "Enjoy your day—today."

An Awareness Mantra

One of the keenest senses of awareness I've ever seen was in one of my patients who's about eighty years old. From the moment I met him, I was struck by his calmness and sense of peace. He was a light. He worked as a volunteer at my hospital and was always very open and friendly to everyone he met. Then one day he ended up with sciatica and became my patient. As I worked with him, I was impressed by how he handled the pain and adversity. Finally I asked him why he was so happy. He was initially hesitant in responding but two weeks later he sent me an email with what he thought were the key ingredients in enjoying his life. His mantra was:

I am whole and powerful.
I am loving and harmonious.
I am forgiving and happy.
I am at peace.

I thought this mantra was great. I tried to memorize it and use it but it just wouldn't stick in my head.

About a year later, the light came on. I was having a disagreement with my wife and was certainly not at peace. I was angry and couldn't let it go. I was also frustrated with myself because, intellectually, I knew I had to let it go. After all, I write about and teach these concepts. I remembered my patient's mantra, and all of a sudden I thought of the connection between the words in each sentence.

- If you are whole, you don't have to spend energy trying to obtain things to make you whole. The result is power to live your life.
- Love is often described as absence of fear. Harmony is one significant result.
- It's not possible to be happy without forgiveness.
- You will not be at peace unless all of the above are present.

Now I have figured out how, through the awareness model, to work backwards through this mantra. Whenever I become aware that I am not at peace, I mentally go through each line to see where I am lacking. Am I not being forgiving? Is something making me feel that I'm not whole? Usually I can quickly see what's disrupting my peace of mind. The next steps may take a while, but at least I know where to go.

Most of my chronic pain patients are not at peace. There are many reasons for this, one of which is lack of forgiveness. Forgiveness in the context of chronic pain is extremely difficult. Many years ago I met a patient who had chronic pain throughout her body, which she'd experienced for over five years. I was struck by how angry she was. She'd been in a car accident and had suffered several major fractures. All of them had healed, but she was still experiencing severe pain. From my orthopedic perspective, there was nothing surgically that could be done to alleviate the pain. She was very upset and openly angry with me. As the conversation went on I learned some details about the accident. She'd been driving her car down a two-lane highway when a drunk driver in a semi-truck crossed over into her lane and hit her head-on. She was completely right in her anger; however, as justified as she was, this chronic anger was destroying her life. Who knows how much effect it was having on her perception of the pain? Almost by definition, one cannot be happy without forgiveness.

In terms of love and harmony, it's very difficult for a chronic pain patient to overcome their fear in order to reach a loving state. Once a patient suffers a significant injury, there's a tremendous amount of fear-related anxiety regarding how, if, and when it will be solved. This is particularly a problem with spinal pain as even the simplest injuries in this area can be very painful. As discussed, the medical profession may not give you clear direction regarding treatment and prognosis. The anxiety becomes overwhelming. It's the antithesis of love and harmony.

I don't know what percentage of people feel less than whole, but I do know that society has a vested interest in convincing you that something's missing. The marketing world implies that you would feel complete if you had a better house, job, spouse, etc. Being in chronic pain is several magnitudes worse. You don't feel whole. You feel your life would be much better without the pain. I do agree with that notion to a point; however, most of us probably didn't feel completely whole before the pain started, and the pain is accentuating any problems.

There's a common belief that "if my circumstances were better, I would be a happier person." This is a flawed concept. It's a barrier to feeling whole. Another way of saying this would be, "If I had less stress in my life, I would be happier." You then begin to spend a lot of time and energy avoiding stress. Instead of embracing new ideas and challenges, you go into a defensive mode. Avoiding stress becomes the ultimate stress. By the way, how are you going to avoid your pain?

Try flipping the paradigm 180 degrees. You *do* have choices when it comes to practicing forgiveness, living your life based on love, and becoming whole. You can choose not to be a victim and live your life in peace. Once you make those choices you'll get to a place where you're creating your own reality on your own terms. You'll have the wherewithal to plug the negative energy drains. It just cannot work the other way around.

FINAL THOUGHTS

Practicing awareness is the first step in reprogramming your brain. It's the easiest technique to explain and the most difficult to consistently use. For me, there's one thing to remember above all: spend as much time as possible doing "active meditation," being fully aware of every stimulus coming into your brain. In other words, try to live your life in the first level of environmental awareness. When you wander into the second level of emotional awareness, just watch your emotions pass by and then pull yourself back into seeing, hearing, and feeling, as quickly as possible.

The third level, that of "the story," is the most difficult for me personally. Once I am sucked into that level, it's hard for me to pull myself back into active meditation although I do think it's possible for someone a little more enlightened than myself. I usually have to use extra tools, such as writing or visualization, to get back on the ground.

Remember that in the fourth level, ingrained patterns, you don't know you're in it without help. With these behaviors, it's impossible to see your real self through your own eyes; it's just the way you are. This is where additional resources such as psychologists, good friends, spouses, children, and seminars have to be utilized.

By the way, becoming aware of everyone and everything around you is much more interesting and enjoyable than merely expressing and reinforcing your own views on life day in and day out. Open yourself up to the world! The possibilities are infinite.

CHAPTER 9
Solving Stress, the Homework

The more time I spend on the DOCC project, the more I realize that almost all my patients who've become pain-free have directed their efforts on their own. I move very quickly in clinic and am always frustrated that I don't have more time to spend with my patients. My role in their rehabilitation has been mostly as a coach and guide. But now I see that a coach/guide is in fact what they need, not someone directing their every move. Their own commitment to the program is the main predictor of success.

In this chapter I've provided "homework" exercises I developed by taking note of my patients' successes. It's my hope that you can achieve the same kind of success using these tools. It's important not only to engage in learning to use the tools, but also to take your time with each phase—*never rush*. Remember, behind you is a lifetime of developing your current ways of behaving. It will take consistent repetition to establish new neurological pathways that bypass your pain, anxiety, and frustration.

Although you'll notice some changes in yourself within the first few weeks or months of doing the program, in my experience, this sequence requires a twelve-to-eighteen-month effort to obtain the full benefit. You'll be practicing many of the new behaviors for the rest of your life.

This chapter is essentially an overview of what we've learned so far, with more detailed exercises that you can use to create your new life. As you'll recall from earlier chapters, to better cope with chronic pain and improve your life, it's critical first to calm down your nervous system. Once it's more calm, you can start taking steps to become more functional and active. The strategies are:

- Education
  - Understand every variable that affects pain perception
- Sleep
- Medication management
  - Pain
  - Anxiety
  - Sleep
- Stress management
  - Desensitizing and reprogramming your nervous system
    ~ Anger
    ~ Anxiety
- Goal Setting
  - Getting your brain re-focused on the future

The process is divided into five stages, each of which has five steps. It's crucial to carve time out of your daily life for each of these stages. Schedule this time as you would anything else in your life that takes priority. What else is more important? Your chronic pain permeates every part of your existence and has a devastating effect on your family.

Don't hurry through these stages, but also don't stop until you are done. Plan on eight to ten weeks per stage. Treat each stage as subject matter that must be mastered. If you fully engage, the majority of what you understand about stress management will be different a year from now. Here's how it breaks down:

Stage I: Address Anxiety
Stage II: Deal with Anger

Stage III: Go From Reactive to Creative
Stage IV: Take Back Your Life
Stage V: Live a Full, Rich Life

STAGE I: ADDRESS ANXIETY

Stage I focuses on anxiety and learning about the complexity of the pain experience. By educating yourself and taking action, you'll probably notice some significant changes in your pain levels and mood within the first four weeks. You may feel a sense of satisfaction, which is a normal reaction—you should be proud of the work you've done so far. Keep going, though; while you may feel better already, know that it takes months for your brain and soft tissues to heal.

Goals

Education

- Understand your diagnosis, which stems from one or more of these three possibilities: 1) structural abnormalities, 2) soft tissue pain, or 3) the Mind Body Syndrome (MBS).
- Identify which of your symptoms might be from MBS.
- Learn the DOCC framework.

Sleep

- Improve by at least 50%, which will usually require medication(s).

Central Nervous System

- Learn about the formation of neurological pathways.
- Begin the "reprogramming process."
- Focus on anxiety and its relationship to pain.

Medications

- Adjust so as to experience: 1) decreased pain, 2) decreased anxiety, and 3) improved sleep.

- Do NOT try to wean off any meds—the goal at this point is to stabilize them.

Goal Setting
- N/A in this phase

Rehabilitation
- Learn basic spine mechanics/anatomy: the book *Eight Steps to a Pain Free Back,* by Esther Gokhale,[1] is an excellent resource.
- Attend "back school" if available (an educational program about back care).
- Hold off on physical therapy until your central nervous system begins to "calm down."
- Join a gym and engage in light training with weights.

Five Steps
Step 1: Nail Down Your Diagnosis

It's critical that you feel comfortable with the diagnosis of your source of pain, which you are likely already investigating with your doctors. If there's a structural problem that's solvable with surgery, the surgery needs to be performed in the context of shared decision making.

In my opinion, over half of the spine surgery performed today should never have been done. What many surgeons define as a "structural" injury is simply normal aging anatomy. For instance, disc degeneration is not a disease and not a reason to perform surgery. If you have a lingering question about whether something is being missed, it's very difficult to move forward with your healing. But remember, for most patients with significant low back pain there is NOT an identifiable source.

Part of identifying your diagnosis is learning about the Mind Body Syndrome. Chronic pain is, essentially, a common symptom of MBS. MBS is extremely treatable; that's why the exercises in this book are so effective. At some point it's like flipping a light switch; when the pain goes away, it goes away—along with many other symptoms.

Unlearn Your Pain, by Howard Schubiner, is a terrific resource for familiarizing yourself with MBS. Chapter 5 of that book includes a self-test to help you see which of your symptoms might be MBS. You may think you're only suffering from physical pain, but trust me, there is usually a MBS component. There is a link to that chapter on www.back-in-control.com.

Step 2: You Are Not Your Thoughts

When you're in chronic pain, your brain lays down pain pathways in a way that's similar to what it does when you learn how to ride a bicycle. But where constant pain is concerned, these neurological circuits are developed along with associated negative thinking that's etched into your neurology.

This is not a typical psychological problem, so traditional psychological approaches do not work. The most effective strategy for "unlearning" the skill of learned pain pathways is via "reprogramming." Writing is the foundation of the reprogramming process.

"You are not your thoughts." Philosophers have taught this concept for a couple thousand years. It's a central part of the DOCC program. It's a simple idea but can be difficult to grasp: even though you might know intellectually that your thoughts don't make up your identity, it certainly may seem like they do.

If you experience anxiety-producing thoughts, they become stronger over time, and if you suppress them they become much worse. The only effective way to deal with these thoughts is to detach from them.

Free Writing

The first thing I have my patients in chronic pain do is to simply start writing down their negative thoughts and then immediately destroy the piece of paper. I call this technique "free writing." Discarding the paper allows you to write with complete freedom. This process connects the *space* between you and the paper with vision and touch. With repetition this separation becomes your new reality.

Free writing is a practice every human being should do on a regular basis from the time they are able to write. It's not about psychology; it's about reprogramming your nervous system. Negative thoughts are a universal part of the human experience; no one escapes the neural circuits they produce. Some are just better at hiding them from themselves and others.

These negative circuits result in deep suffering, and there's always a price to pay if you try to control them. The more despicable and bizarre the thoughts you can release by writing them down are, the more effective the process. Those are the thoughts that require the most emotional energy to suppress. Consider it a task you'll do regularly for the rest of your life, like brushing your teeth or bathing. It's "mental hygiene."

I've found that in doing the writing exercises, some of my patients have a tendency to write multiple times per day with the idea that if enough thoughts are "captured" and processed, life will be better. But this exercise is *not* about recording your thoughts; it's about *letting them go*. If you feel the urge to capture your thoughts, remember that the point of this method is to detach from what's in your mind, not control it.

As you write down your thoughts, remember to toss the paper out right away. This will help you to write without any inhibitions. A few other pointers for the writing exercises:

- Don't just write *about* the thoughts; write down your actual thoughts. The darker the thoughts, the more effective the process, since they're the ones that take the most unconscious energy to contain.
- Write once or twice a day for fifteen to thirty minutes per session.

- Handwrite. Research has shown that a large part of the brain is activated when you write on paper.[2] I don't know how effective typing on a computer might be in comparison.
- Do not try to "journal" or keep these writings; it's counter-productive. Also, note that writing down positive alternatives, etc. is a different type of exercise.
- Write in the free-flow format for a couple of weeks and then start to engage in the Feeling Good format described below.

Your journey to a pain-free life will begin the day you commit to writing. It won't start until then.

The Feeling Good Format
- Once you're in the habit of free writing, read the first third of David Burns's book, *Feeling Good*.
- Then, in addition to free writing, write in Burns "three-column" format.
- Continue to destroy ALL of your writing immediately (including the three-column format writing).

Note, David Burns's three-column format represents the phases of reprogramming: 1) awareness, 2) detachment, and 3) establishing new circuits. Also note that *Feeling Good* is a great resource on its own, but not nearly as effective without the writing exercises.

The main reason I have patients get in the habit of free writing before doing the three-column work is that the book is so interesting it will distract you from the writing. Once you've settled into the writing exercises, read *Feeling Good* in its entirety. It outlines a remarkably helpful and insightful set of tools. This book is what single-handedly pulled me out of a very deep hole.

Step 3: Neurological Pathways—Not Psychology

To better understand neurological pathways, do the following:

- Read the book *The Talent Code* by Dan Coyle.[3] He's a wonderful writer who elucidates how genius is formed in athletes, musicians, and artists, linking it to recent neuroscientific research. Coyle discusses how the brain lays down a substance called myelin, which insulates the pathways of skill, making them stronger. The same principles seem to apply to pain, anxiety, and the associated frustrations.

- Re-read the text about the "White Bear" study described in Chapter 1, performed by Daniel Wegner. Wegner's experiment demonstrated that when you try not to think about something, you'll think about it more. That's why the darker the thoughts you can get down on paper, the more effective the writing process.

- Consider Wegner's essay, "The Seed of Our Undoing,"[4] in which he explains that each of us has within us the key to our own downfall. The "seed" in this case is trying to control/suppress our thoughts, which he calls the "ironic effect." When we try not to think about something we think about it more and access the thoughts more quickly. Doing the opposite—i.e., trying to think about something—causes us to think about it less. Simply writing or saying "unthinkable" thoughts negates this "ironic effect." This strategy is the foundation of the whole mental health component of the DOCC program.

A conversation that I frequently have with my patients in clinic starts like this: "Think about someone you strongly dislike. You don't have to say his or her name, but get a clear picture of that person." I give them a few seconds and then they usually nod yes, they have it. "You're being judgmental. Right?" Again they'll nod yes. "Now you've realized that being judgmental is taking away from the quality of your life and you don't want to be that way anymore, so you decide not to be judgmental when you meet or think about this person."

Withholding judgment might seem like the best way to go, but here's what just happened: if the patient continued to be judgmental they would continue to suffer. On the flip side, if you try to be positive and convince yourself to like this person, it's much worse. "Not being judgmental" really reinforces your judgmental neurological pathways. Patients immediately see the problem. So what do you do?

Write the actual judgmental thoughts down!! The more graphically you can write them down the more effective the exercise. You cannot get rid of those circuits but detaching from them means that they are no longer running the show. When you do interact with the person, you don't have to like them. In fact you may continue to dislike them. However, you can now deal with whatever issue is at hand based just on its merit. In other words, you can enter each interaction with that person free of any prejudice or assumptions, opening yourself to the possibility of developing a meaningful relationship. With labels in place there are *no* possibilities. You don't like being labeled a "chronic pain patient." Why should other people you come in contact with enjoy your labels on them? Finally, your interaction with others is a direct reflection on your interaction with yourself. The more peaceful and content you are with yourself, the easier your interactions with others will be (and vice versa). Let it ALL go: your judgments/labels of yourself *and* others—it makes for a better life.

Step 4: Get Some Sleep

Sleep is *number one* in the rehabilitation process. The only reason I put calming down the nervous system ahead of sleep in this section is that the calming tools will also help you sleep. *None* of the DOCC principles will be effective if you are not getting seven or eight hours of restful sleep per night. Certain medication combinations will allow you to sleep regardless of your pain levels. Not one major decision regarding your spine care should be made until you feel rested during the day. Make it your responsibility to work with your primary care physician to get a restful night's sleep on a regular basis.

Step 5: DOCC Principles and the Mind Body Syndrome

I feel that the main contribution the DOCC program makes to the treatment of chronic pain is that it points out the links between pain, anxiety, and anger. These are then connected to the idea of neurological pathways instead of psychology, with a focus on creating alternate pathways. The more you understand these relationships, the more effectively you'll be able to design your own program for developing a rich, full, and pain-free life.

In the Mind Body Syndrome, a traumatic event or intense anger can establish a real, learned pain pathway that can be reactivated at any time. Recall from Chapter 7 the man whose pain was triggered by the sound of helicopters (which he'd heard in Vietnam when he had his initial injury) even though doctors could find nothing wrong with him. Even when there's no tissue damage in the body, such as a tumor, a fracture, or an infection, a learned pathway can cause real physical pain.

The DOCC model helps you work through MBS by introducing new, alternative neurological pathways into your daily existence.

There is no specific magic to the DOCC model. It's just a framework that organizes well-established chronic pain and spine care concepts. Through this program, you will begin to see your health care providers as resources and coaches instead of relying on them entirely for your rehab. You'll be given the tools to organize your thinking and healthcare so that you can take charge of getting better. As you regain control your frustrations will abate, which will enable you to reconnect with the essence of who you really are.

The reason I'm presenting this material in so many different ways and in such detail is that the concepts are the opposite of what most of us have been taught about how to manage pain and stress. It's important to deepen your understanding of the factors that affect your perception of pain and equally important to understand the Mind Body Syndrome in detail. Pain is just one of many symptoms of this syndrome. Here's how to learn the principles:

- Utilize the website www.back-in-control.com as a resource (updated weekly). The whole website is structured around this chapter. Many patient success stories and informational videos are posted on the site.
- Read *Unlearn Your Pain* and take Dr. Schubiner's test to see what other components of MBS apply to your situation (everyone has some of these symptoms).

My patients' success is proportional to the degree of their involvement and commitment. Over time I have observed a consistent improvement in their pain and quality of life. Caring for those of my patients in chronic pain has become the most rewarding and enjoyable aspect of my practice.

I never would have been so presumptuous with these statements even six months ago. But the results I've seen have been dramatic. I have never seen anyone fully engage in the program and not get better—it's only a matter of time.

More About Writing

Again, writing down negative thoughts, or "free writing," is an extremely effective way of separating yourself from those thoughts. After all, a thought is just a series of connections between neurons within your brain; there is no substance to it. None. However, when your body secretes chemicals in response to this thought, it seems like it's real and a part of your identity. Your goal is to bring the troublesome thought to life as vividly as possible so you can then process it. Again, three events occur when you write down such a thought: 1) you're creating a "space" between yourself and that thought, 2) you're associating that space with vision and touch, which creates a new and different neurologic pathway, and 3) you're detaching from the spinning circuits in your mind.

For instance, if you write down, "My daughter is disrespectful," you've created a space between her behavior and your reaction. You've enabled yourself to see the effect that the thought has on you and your relationship with her. You might notice that you've labeled her. In addition, your eyes read the words and the thought goes back into your brain on a different circuit. You've also felt your pen write the words, so the thought is associated with a sense of touch. Some advocate saying the thought out loud, which would go back into your brain through your auditory system. The net effect is that you have dramatically heightened your awareness of the offending thought or pattern of thoughts. If you just tried to rationalize the upsetting thoughts in your head, they would only spin faster.

I have personally practiced variations of this method for many years. Doing so was instrumental in finally pulling me out of a severe depression. I also had the support of a psychologist and psychiatrist, which I think can be extremely helpful for many if not most people. But the core of the process was the discipline of writing on an almost daily basis.

The nervous system is extremely complex; a small percentage of connections in the brain result in thoughts that are bizarre, crazy, despicable, unspeakable, and just simply unacceptable at every level. However, they are just thoughts.

The writing process is not a quick fix. I've had patients come back disappointed that they didn't have more immediate results. The problem in this scenario is that they were writing with an agenda, with the goal of "fixing" themselves or getting rid of the pain. The purpose of this kind of writing is to start connecting to yourself—that is all. You cannot "fix" your brain; you can only implement strategies that allow it to heal.

In order to get the most out of the writing process, it's important to depersonalize it. Remember, you're using mechanical means to deal with irrational circuits. Everyone experiences these circuits, and though some people are better at covering them up than others, they always surface in some way.

Some patients tell me that the writing process is disturbing. I then know they have really engaged in the activity. If you don't begin to uncover some uncomfortable emotions, you haven't really committed to it. I've been at this long enough to know that if someone tells me how great life is on the first follow-up visit, they haven't started writing.

I recently had a patient who'd successfully undergone a successful disc excision that resulted in complete relief of her leg pain. But even though the surgery came out well, she still had a lot of vocational issues to deal with and was appropriately angry. She initially didn't see or acknowledge her anger, so several weeks after the surgery I finally convinced her to begin writing. She pursued it with a vengeance and even consented to see the pain psychologist I work with. She seemed to be doing well with both the stress-related issues and her spine, but then it all came to a halt. When I asked her how the writing was going about three months after surgery she replied, "I stopped. First I realized that I was an angry person. Then, as I kept writing, I started to feel depressed. I'd rather be angry than depressed." I then had a very circular conversation with her for about twenty minutes before I finally gave up. I don't know what happened to her after that.

It was during this interaction a couple of years ago that I realized how strong anger was in combating anxiety. While you in the midst of feeling angry you feel very little if any anxiety. I also feel that anxiety also drives depression. In the short term he did feel more anxiety/depression. However long-term he will have missed the opportunity to connect with himself with the potential of living a more rich and full life.

I used the *Feeling Good* book as a personal resource for many years until I finally realized in 1997 that I could also use it in my practice. I liked using the book clinically because it was much faster than trying to get someone in to see a pain psychologist. It was a tool patients could use almost immediately, and they often did so aggressively. Burns's book was the entire mental health component of the DOCC project for many years.

The initial goal of the DOCC project was to help patients live with their pain, but I was pleasantly surprised to hear that in many cases the pain would go away completely.

It was puzzling to me, though, why some patients would respond so much better than others. It eventually became clear that the patients who did well were the ones who participated wholeheartedly in the writing process, so I placed even more emphasis on the importance of writing.

Patients who **commit** to a daily writing process based on the suggestions in *Feeling Good* **always** have a significant, if not dramatic, response. The results have been consistent. If you only educate yourself about the DOCC concepts without doing any writing, it can be somewhat counter-productive. By just reading about reha- bilitation, you take in a lot of great advice, but sometimes that only gives you more ammunition to think about your issues and keep the anxiety-producing thoughts in your head spinning.

Many patients do the program for a few months and then lose interest, as they want quicker results. Some quit because they are doing so much better than before. However, I feel that they're missing a huge opportunity to live life at a level they haven't yet comprehended. Reprogramming the nervous system takes repe- tition over an extended period of time. In fact, at some level it really shouldn't ever stop.

The first third of *Feeling Good* describes in detail how cogni- tive behavioral therapy works. Burns's ten "errors in thinking," which we discussed earlier in this book, cover the range of nega- tive thinking. They include:

- "Should" thinking
- Catastrophizing

- Labeling
- Minimizing the positive
- Emphasizing the negative

He then presents the "three-column" technique, which is essentially the only cognitive behavioral method I used for over eight years. It's a highly effective way to process stress.

In the three-column technique, you create three columns on a piece of paper. In the first column you write down your "ANT," which stands for "automatic negative thought." This step increases the awareness of disruptive thoughts. In the second column, you write down the "error in thinking" that the thought represents. As you consider the error, analyze the thought, and see the effect it's having on your peace of mind, the thought's power diminishes. This helps you to detach from it. In the third column you write down the more rational thought. The more specific you are, the better. Putting this subsequent thought in writing helps you to burn a new, healthier circuit in your mind.

For example, imagine your son flunked a test at school. Your first response might be, "He's lazy and stupid." Using the three-column technique, you'd write those thoughts down in the first column. In the second column you'd note that your thoughts were "labeling," "catastrophizing," and "overgeneraliz- ing." In the third column you might write, "My son just flunked a test. I wonder why. Is he being bullied at school? Could he be depressed? I need to try to find out what's going on."

Note that what you've done is different from positive think- ing. With positive thinking, you would've written, "He isn't lazy. He's my son and I love him," and that might be it. Except, without writing a more specific rational response, your thoughts might start to spin around. By the time you actually talked to him, you probably wouldn't be in a great frame of mind.

The writing process takes daily commitment and discipline. Again, the changes you're trying to effect in your nervous system only occur with repetition. However, I've noticed that change usually happens quickly if a person truly engages. Within three to four weeks of ten to twenty minutes of daily writing, my patients will come in quite enthusiastic about the effects they're feeling. And fifteen years after I started, *I'm* still writing. My wife can tell within a few days if I temporarily stop; my reactivity tends to increase. I feel that the repro-gramming process is a lifetime commitment. It's "neurological maintenance."

Resources for Stage I

The Talent Code, by Dan Coyle
Feeling Good, by David Burns
Eight Steps to a Pain-Free Back, by Esther Gokhale
Unlearn Your Pain, by Howard Schubiner, M.D.

Checklist for Moving to Stage II:

- Understand the source of your pain, including which of your symptoms might be attributable to the Mind Body Syndrome.
  - Be familiar with the concepts in *Unlearn Your Pain*
- Finished *The Talent Code.*
- Finished the first third of *Feeling Good.*
  - Actively engaged in fifteen to thirty minutes of writing daily, including the free writing of negative thoughts and the three-column technique.
- Sleep is modestly improved.
- Understand basic spine mechanics either through a detailed book or a back school.
- Be lightly working out in a gym three to five hours per week.

Spend at least six to eight weeks on Stage I. Don't try to rush through any of these stages. It takes repetition for the process to be effective.

Stage II: Deal with Anger

Stage II is about anger. Although it's only the second of five phases, it's the one that will determine whether you can truly move on or remain mired in the past. At some point during the process of working through your anger, your pain will begin to decrease significantly. Sometimes it happens quickly.

By definition, being in chronic pain means you will feel legitimately angry. Letting go of that anger is the "continental divide" of chronic pain. If you don't think you're angry in the presence of unrelenting pain, you're just not connected to it. It's normal to deny anger—after all, most of us really hate feeling angry. However, recognizing your anger and taking steps to defuse it is the only way to start your new life.

Goals

Education
- Resolve any questions about surgery, and either undergo a procedure or not.
- Learn more about the Mind Body Syndrome

Sleep
- Full night's sleep
- Usually still need meds

Central Nervous System
- Focus is on anger, which is driven by pain
- Understand how anger both masks and fuels anxiety
- Recognize and acknowledge your own victim role
- Consider psychological support

Medications
- Continue to stabilize them
- Weaning off is still not a priority

Goal Setting
- N/A in this phase

Rehabilitation
- Begin physical therapy
- Continue at the gym—light weight training
- Increase aerobic activity–walking, swimming, etc.

Five Steps
Step 1: Understand the Interaction Between
Pain, Anxiety, and Anger

In this step we focus on understanding how pain, anxiety, and anger relate. (Note: this is a review of concepts we discussed earlier in the book that you can use as part of the homework process.)

- Not being in pain is a basic human need, such as the need for air, food, or water. When this need isn't met, you feel anxiety.
- Next comes anger over the loss of your ability to resolve the problem (i.e., meet your basic need.)
- Anger makes you feel powerful, which covers the feelings of anxiety, and yet also reinforces your anxiety-producing circuits. It's the turbo-charger that must be turned off.
- You blame yourself or your situation for your predicament; doing so puts you in the victim role.

The circumstance making you feel like a victim may be perceived or real. Examples of perceived victimhood are: a) being cut off in traffic, b) not being invited to a party, or c) not having enough free time. Examples of real victimhood are: a) being physically assaulted/or and robbed, b) being the subject of vicious gossip, or c) being wrongfully imprisoned.

The difference between real and perceived victimhood is that real victimhood is much more difficult to let go of. Chronic pain is REAL victimhood.

Even though you're a real victim (with chronic pain), it's vital to understand the devastating effects that your pain and anger have on your immediate family. When you're chronically angry you cannot see their needs clearly and it's likely that much of your interaction with them is abusive. I strongly advise my patients to never interact with family members if they are angry, and I recommend the same for you.

Step 2: Identify Your Own Victimhood

Use the following tools to get in touch with your victim role:

- Ask yourself, "What person or circumstance is upsetting me?" Be specific.
- Acknowledge that you are blaming that person or situation for making you angry.
- Write or speak out loud to yourself, "I blame [So-and-So or such-and-such] for making me upset."
- Understand that you are now in the victim role, which is a universal feeling: we all experience it.
- Write or speak, "I am allowing myself to be a victim of [see above]."

Differentiate clearly in your own mind whether you are: 1) Being truly victimized or 2) Basing your victimization on a perception that comes from a "story" in your mind. Note how much more difficult it is to process the anger if you've been truly victimized.

Obviously your chronic pain will be high on the list of circumstances that are making you feel like a victim. However, don't let this get in the way of identifying the multitude of other ways you might be playing that role. Anytime you're frustrated or angry you're in victim mode. Whenever you feel angry, instead of blaming someone (or something), take full responsibility. Learn to do the above exercise on a regular basis.

I confess, admitting to my victim status has been the most challenging part of my own journey. I went through a phase where I thought that I'd learned enough about being a victim and that I was "above it." I considered myself enlightened. It was a bad phase of my life.

Step 3: Commit to Stop Being a Victim

Once you get a clear sense of the depth of your anger and victimhood, make a simple decision to not be a victim anymore.

- Write down, "I choose not to be a victim." Date it and put it where you'll see it on a daily basis. Remember that:
  - It's an intellectual choice that needs to be accompanied by reprogramming tools in order to be effective. Your intellect cannot contain the level of frustration associated with being in chronic pain.
  - You will repeatedly fail, and that's okay. Don't stop your efforts.
  - You must commit to being honest with yourself.
- "Do." (Hoffman Process concept)
  - "I will try" is the ultimate victim phrase. Write "try" on a piece of paper, cross it out, and hang it on your refrigerator.
  - Write "Do" on another piece of paper and hang it on your bathroom mirror.

I made the choice to stop being a victim on Mother's Day 2002. It's still a daily challenge, but my life took a dramatic turn out of the Abyss that day.

Step 4: Take Off Your Disguises

None of us like the idea that we might be acting like victims. We don't even like the word, and there are an infinite number of ways to disguise it. Here a few of my personal favorite methods:

- Being "right"
- Feeling sorry for myself
- Suppressing thoughts

- Disassociating—closing the door on the past
- Adopting an identity of being "cool and calm"
- Being perfectionist/judgmental
- Holding onto high ideals/standards
- Having strong opinions

My "go to" one is "I'm frustrated." I did not realize for many years that frustration and anger were essentially the same word. My list would truly fill a thick book, as this may be my most highly evolved life skill. Write down the disguises you may be using. This exercise will provide you with better awareness of who you are. Save the list.

Step 5: Accept and Forgive

The forgiveness step is an individual, personal process. Many books have been written on the subject over the centuries. The book that's been the most effective for my patients and me is *Forgive for Good,* by Fred Luskin.[5] Luskin, director of the Stanford University Forgiveness Project, has conducted four major research projects on this topic. He discusses the nature of true forgiveness and provides steps for achieving it. *Forgive for Good* was pointed out to me by a patient and has had a major impact on my patients' pain and quality of life. It was when this book entered the DOCC project that my patients began to experience a remarkable decrease in their pain. I also realized how deep a connection that pain has with anger.

Somewhere in the midst of working through deep anger issues—a process that, by necessity, includes acceptance and forgiveness—chronic pain often diminishes or even disappears. Conversely if you think about it in terms of circuits and connections it is essentially impossible to decrease your pain without truly letting of your legitimate anger.

Forgiveness and acceptance are difficult for me, personally, but I know that they're crucial. In my experience, it helps for me to keep in mind a few strategies that DON'T work:

- Positive thinking
- Denial, "intellectual" rather than heartfelt forgiveness and acceptance
- Adherence to extreme belief systems

Positive Thinking

Throughout this book, I've stressed the fact that positive thinking is not an effective way to deal with life's issues, including chronic pain. And here again, I'd like to emphasize that positive thinking is another way of suppressing negative thinking. It doesn't work to suppress your feelings of anger and rage against the person or situation that has treated you poorly; first you have to experience the feelings. You can't "think" your way out of anger by trying to have positive thoughts about whoever has done you wrong. Only by truly forgiving him or her can you move forward.

Part of not resorting to positive thinking is accepting at a very deep emotional level that the pain you feel today is the pain you will have, in some form, for the rest of your life. Chronic pain can and will outlast you. Acceptance of this fact is a major starting point in dealing with your chronic pain-related stress reactions. If you are obsessed with having your pain magically disappear, then your nervous system will focus on the pain even more. The idea is to get yourself functional and not be a *victim* of your pain.

Letting go of positive thinking also involves regaining perspective on your entire life. Many people in chronic pain get caught up in thoughts like, "Someday the doctor will fix me and my life will be perfect." But when I ask my patients (most of whom are between the ages of thirty-five and fifty-five), "How are you going to live the next thirty or forty or fifty years with this pain?" they wake right up. They've usually been bounced around the medical system without any coordinated plan or any control. Many, if not most, are so caught up in their immediate anger that they don't realize they need to look at their lives differently. You cannot "positively think" yourself out of a noxious physical sensation.

One patient that I treated was clearly a positive thinker, and unfortunately, from what I could see, his outlook hindered rather than helped his situation. Alan was a fifty-five-year-old business-man who started having various orthopedic procedures at age forty. His first spine operation was a laminectomy performed about ten years earlier just for back pain. A year later a fusion was done between the fourth and fifth vertebrae for ongoing low back pain. Over a nine-year period, his spine dramatically broke down above and below the fusion. By the time he saw me he was tilted forward about 30 degrees and tilted to his right side about 40 degrees. He had to use a walker much of the time. In the interim he had also had both hips replaced, four knee arthroscopies, and both shoulders scoped. In addition to being crooked, he felt pain throughout his whole body. In other words, he'd had multiple operations and was in bad physical shape and yet, surprisingly, on his initial intake questionnaire he rated himself as a zero on a scale of ten regarding anxiety, depression, and irritability.

I performed a major surgery through Alan's stomach, during which I inserted four cages with bone graft to wedge open and correct the deformity. I then turned him over and inserted rods from his second lumbar vertebra to his pelvis. I was success-ful in restoring him to a nearly normal posture and he was extremely grateful.

Even though Alan's posture was restored, he still faced recov-ery, as well as chronic pain in other areas of his body. He contin-ued not to acknowledge any stress issues, though, and I could not crack his armor. It was clear to me how frustrated he was with all of his orthopedic limitations at so early an age, but I couldn't persuade him to do any writing or engage with the pain psychol-ogist that I work with. About once every four visits he would get close to exploding, but then stuff it. I found it interesting that despite his pain, he had an extraordinarily engaging personality and was seemingly happy. There was always a big smile on his face and I enjoyed his visits. All I could surmise was that he was very skilled at suppressing his anxiety.

I never did get through to Alan. He continued to experience chronic pain and, shortly after I was done seeing him, underwent a total knee replacement.

If you are in chronic pain and haven't been given any answers or direction from the medical establishment but really, truly, do not feel any anger, put on your gloves and start digging through your veneer of positive thinking.

Extreme Belief Systems

Common mechanisms used to suppress anxiety are rigid thinking, control, and over-dependence on structure. These methods become apparent when anyone tries to control people and circumstances at home and work so they don't have to feel any anxiety about future outcomes.

Extreme belief systems fall into this category, which can be in almost any arena; examples are religion, politics, and nationalism. In this scenario, you become attached to being "right." What you may not realize, though, is that this attachment is really thinly disguised anger, even if you don't consciously feel angry. Watch your reaction when someone disagrees with or questions your belief system; it will be an angry one. Someone merely disagreed with you; you weren't physically threatened or harmed. Why would you become so reactive?

I have deep respect for any person's religious beliefs—that's not the issue. It's the consequences when you hide behind these systems that concerns me.

Among the patients I've seen who cede the solution for their chronic pain to a rigid religious code, I've never witnessed one improve their life, function, or pain. I've tried everything from a full-on frontal assault to using logic, but I cannot get through.

One such case was Paul, a forty-year old laborer who'd injured his back about ten years earlier. His chief complaint was low back pain and he also had some left leg pain. Paul weighed well over three hundred and fifty pounds and was markedly out of shape. Against my better instincts I performed a small operation to remove a bone spur from his right L4 nerve root. I'd made it clear that I didn't have any hope that this procedure would decrease his back pain. His leg pain, however, seemed to resolve a little after the procedure. His back pain continued unabated and he remained severely disabled.

Paul was steadfast in feeling that his church and religious beliefs were the solution to his problems. We had every type of conversation you could imagine about him hiding his issues behind his religion. I would not have had those conversations except his pain level kept escalating and he demanded more medications. I tried over the course of two years to persuade him to engage in some type of self-awareness work, with no success. At one point he received a disability settlement/pension and bought a small farm to live on—which I thought would calm him down a little—but it didn't seem to help.

Finally, one day in the middle of a busy clinic he stood up and started to scream at me at the top of his lungs, "F--- you! F---ing doctors!! You don't know what the f--- you're doing!" He would not stop and made a move as if to hit me. Then he walked through my full waiting room screaming. Two weeks later he shot himself.

I felt, and still feel, a lot of compassion for Paul. I did understand his frustration but I just couldn't break through his intellectual defenses. And as much as I encouraged him, he wouldn't see a psychiatrist.

A deep spiritual connection to yourself and a higher power can be critical to healing. I fully support developing a deep, genuine faith, and many of my patients have had great success with the support of their religious leaders and fellow believers. However any religious belief system that is critical of one's self or others, such as the one that Paul followed, is incredibly damaging. This is one kind of situation where I cannot penetrate a patient's certainty and have to let go—quickly.

Intellectual Forgiveness versus True Acceptance

I was raised in a fundamentalist church that taught forgiveness is the essence of life. Yet at the same time many, if not most, religious cultures are intolerant of other belief systems. I still have many friends in the church community and I have a lot of respect for faith. But how can you be truly forgiving and judgmental at the same time? True forgiveness is a critical part of living a full, rich life connected to your family and friends; that said, I know that reaching that point at an emotional level is very challenging.

For me, the tragedy of Paul's story is that I know from our conversations that he thought forgiveness was important. He knew that he needed to forgive the medical system for any way in which he felt mistreated. For Paul to get to that point, though, he would have had to first experience the full depth of his anger and rage and then process it using some of the methods I've already suggested. If you don't experience your anger, it will continue to simmer beneath the surface of any attempts you make at forgiveness; you won't be coming from a place of genuine peace.

Some consider certain acts unforgivable. (Imagine, for example, surgery that disables you for life.) I once would've agreed with that notion. In the past, I felt that forgiving certain deeds would be like denying they had happened. And I still think that there's a fine line between forgiveness/acceptance and denial. I now realize, however, that it's critical to forgive regardless of the extent of the misdeed.

Luskin points out that forgiveness is only for you; it has nothing to do with the perpetrator. And it has to be real, deep forgiveness. Intellectually forgiving someone or something in your past has a positive effect, but it only scratches the surface compared to really digging in, feeling, and creating alternate, forgiving neurologic pathways.

Resources for Stage II:

- *Forgive for Good,* by Dr. Fred Luskin
- *Back in Control,* Anxiety/Anger chapter
- Consultation with a pain psychologist
- Support from a religious or spiritual leader

Checklist for Moving to Stage III:

- Continue to free write and also write in the Feeling Good three-column format.
- Finish reading and engaging in the tools from *Forgive for Good.*
- Full acceptance of your victim role
- Sleep should be seven to eight hours per night—with or without meds.
- Physical therapy is completed.
- Light workouts in the gym three to five hours per week, with weights
- Completed all of the above five steps—it's not possible to effectively move into Stage III without taking full responsibility for your frustrations and anger.
- Give yourself at least eight to ten weeks on this phase—or as much time as you need. This phase seems to have the most impact on decreasing pain.

STAGE III: GO FROM REACTIVE TO CREATIVE

Picture yourself climbing out of a deep crevasse, standing up, and looking around. The ground you stand on represents the life you had before you fell into the abyss of chronic pain. You've been in the crevasse for so long that it's difficult to remember your former life. This phase is where you begin to connect with your true self. This section is about *awareness.*

Goals

Education
- Learn four levels of awareness: 1) environmental, 2) emotional, 3) "the story," and 4) ingrained patterns.
- Learn to maintain your peace of mind regardless of external circumstances.
- Go deeper into learning about the Mind Body Syndrome and how it applies to your symptoms.

Sleep
- Full night's sleep with minimal or no meds–easier when anger has been successfully addressed

Central Nervous System
- Learn the awareness tools that will calm you.
- Use "active meditation" to reach a baseline awareness.
- Become aware of your "unawareness."
- Understand the power of imagery.

Medications
- Pain meds decreasing
- Anti-anxiety and sleep meds decreasing

Goal Setting
- Reconnect with the best part of your past.
- Begin to re-form your life vision.

Rehabilitation
- Resistance training three to five times per week
- Aerobic conditioning
- Healthy back mechanics integrated into activities of daily living

Five Steps
Step 1: Understand Awareness and Unawareness

Being aware means being fully involved in the present moment. There are numerous time-tested tools for increasing awareness:

- Mindfulness (paying attention), visualization, and meditation
- Actively cultivating your ability to listen and feel

The role of awareness in the neural reprogramming process involves three steps: 1) awareness, 2) detachment, and 3) creating new circuits. As you go through these steps, you will also become "aware of your unawareness," that is, begin to notice when you are not paying attention to the present moment. (Note that the difficulty of this step will become clear only in retrospect as you learn how to be fully aware.)

Four Levels of Awareness

Awareness is a word that's easily tossed around. Most of us feel that we're reasonably aware of what's happening around us. However, as I've traveled on my own journey I've realized that true awareness is a challenge; it's also a humbling process. Getting there can be unsettling, and yet it's also an intensely freeing experience. It's the gateway to a life you have not yet comprehended.

Instead of listening carefully with an open mind, I've spent most of my life imposing my interpretation of reality onto a given situation. I didn't realize that good listening is a learned skill that goes hand in hand with awareness. To heighten my own awareness, it's been helpful for me to conceptualize it at these four levels:

- Environmental
- Emotional
- Judgment/"Stories"
- Ingrained behavioral patterns

Step 2: Environmental Awareness and Active Meditation

We are a goal-oriented society that's focused outward on experiences and accomplishments. We're spending less and less quiet time with ourselves and with those close to us, failing to connect with the current moment. But we do this at our own peril: connecting to the moment at hand is the essence of fully experiencing your life. Here's a way to better connect that I've found immensely useful:

- Learn "active meditation," an excellent method for engaging in what's right in front of you. Active meditation involves choosing to pay attention to one of your senses in particular (I most often use sound or touch). This will help bring you back into the moment when your mind wanders. Spend as much time as you can during the day using your chosen sense to stay in the moment. Begin each day with a commitment to work on staying in that mode.
  - Touch/Feeling
  - Sound/Hearing
  - Breathing
  - Vision
  - Taste

Active meditation is a "go-to" strategy for calming yourself throughout the day.

Step 3: Emotional Awareness

Being emotionally aware means noticing and acknowledging your emotions throughout the day; it's the opposite of suppression. As discussed, suppressing emotions doesn't work. You cannot selectively suppress one of your emotions, and if you try you'll suppress your whole nervous system and diminish your range of emotional experience. Eventually joy will be experienced as just moderately less anxiety, and peacefulness will be felt as less chaos.

Being aware of your emotions includes watching all of them come and go. Here's how:

- As anxiety enters your consciousness, learn to just watch it come in like it's a visitor and then watch it leave. Don't try to shove it out the door; you'll lose that battle. Eventually, you'll train yourself to not react to unpleasant, anxiety-producing thoughts. This is the essence of a meditative practice.

- Become aware of what anger does to you. It's as if a filter or screen is pulled over your eyes and you can see things only through this filter; you also can't receive any input without distortion. As a result, you're completely detached from reality. As I lived much of my life with disguised anger as my baseline, I didn't recognize it for what it was. I was just always "right" and couldn't figure out why people didn't see the power of my arguments. In retrospect, I realize that often I wasn't even on the same topic as the people with whom I disagreed.

- Use active meditation as your baseline; it will sensitize you to the presence of your emotions. Active meditation has made me keenly aware of when my anger switch is flipped on. Because I now know that I can (and do) spend much of my time in a peaceful state of mind—regardless of my external circumstances—it's particularly distressing when I slip out of it. The contrast is brutal. It's humbling to me how deep and strong my "anger circuits" really are.

- Remember that the energy used suppressing negative emotions is the very energy you need to create solutions to your problems.

Step 4: Judgment/"Stories"

"He that is without sin among you, let him first cast a stone." (John 8:7)

We all know this biblical lesson. It tells us to be aware of our judgmental natures. It alerts us to the fact that our "stories" have the power to hold us back. I'll use an example from my profession.

Judgment runs strong in the medical world. That's because the culture of medicine is immersed in "high standards," "high ideals," and perfectionism. Society *demands* perfection from physicians. This demand is manifested in many ways: the legal system's treatment of medicine; lack of help with stress management; lack of mercy for personal mental health issues; and harsh criticism from our mentors. Consequently, as others judge us, we turn idealistic about our own standards of performance and become self-critical. Unfortunately, we're also hard on others around us. This leads to labeling of ourselves as well as anyone we come in contact with. Once you label someone, you can no longer really "see" the essence of who they are. (The same holds true for labeling yourself.)

The work of Epictetus (circa 55-135 CE), a Greek Stoic philosopher who was born a Roman slave, can help us refrain from being judgmental. We know him only from writings by others, especially his student Arian, who testifies that he wrote down as much as he could of his mentor's teachings. Since antiquity, however, the teachings of this former slave have influenced generations of thinkers and his observations are considered the foundation of modern cognitive behavioral therapy. *The Art of Living: Epictetus, A New Interpretation,* by Sharon Lebell,[6] discusses the damaging effects of judgment both of self and of others:

> When we name things correctly, we comprehend them correctly, without adding information or judgments that aren't there. Does someone bathe quickly? Don't say he bathes poorly, but quickly. Name the situation as it is; don't filter it through your judgments.

Does someone drink a lot of wine? Don't say she is a drunk but that she drinks a lot. Unless you possess a comprehensive understanding of her life, how do you know if she is a drunk?

Do not risk being beguiled by appearances and constructing theories and interpretations based on distortions through misnaming. Give your assent only to that what is actually true.

I recommend you read a page or two of *The Art of Living* on a regular basis. A few other tools for you to use:

- Avoiding saying, "he or she is a chronic pain patient." Instead say, "He or she is suffering from pain that is chronic." In this way, you refrain from defining a person by their pain. What is the label you put on yourself? Do you view yourself as a "chronic pain patient"?
- Understand that your stories will become your reality. Your mind works in images and the imagery is powerful. You might notice that any large organization that wishes to convey a certain belief system makes liberal use of images. A film called *Cinema Paradiso*, which I discussed in Chapter 4, will convey to you the power of imagery. It's also a great movie.
- Increase your awareness of the judgments inherent in our world, as well as the depth of anger that underpins our society. What we've been led to believe is a normal baseline attitude is actually very destructive to a personal sense of well-being.

Step 5: Ingrained Behavioral Patterns

Ingrained patterns are "baseline" behaviors that seem normal but are often, in fact, dysfunctional. To get beyond them, engage an outside party to help you see what you cannot see about yourself. Any resistance you feel to that idea is your biggest clue that you need to "look under the hood." Every human struggles with anxiety. Yet instead of just admitting it and helping each other out we spend an enormous amount of energy trying to cover it up.

Our ingrained patterns are challenging to tease out because they represent our basic life overview. It's the way we've always been. One of the biggest paradigm shifts I ever experienced was recognizing that I'd had a great deal of anxiety since I was a very young child being raised in a difficult household. Up until then, that past was simply my only frame of reference. How could I have missed *that* for over thirty years?

Discovering your own ingrained patterns will take an open mind and a concerted effort over a long period of time. I don't see how this can be accomplished on your own. It requires a format where you can receive honest feedback from a mental health professional or other person trained in providing support. After all, if your life outlook has flaws, any attempt to see your patterns will be flawed by definition.

Our ingrained patterns also come into play in the Mind Body Syndrome. In Stage III, continue reading *Unlearn Your Pain*, learning about MBS and its concepts in detail. As many of the physical symptoms described in MBS are caused by our ingrained patterns of behavior and difficulties in coping with stress, start from where you are and work backwards. In other words, first look at your symptoms and then figure out what circumstances might be triggering those pain pathways.

Note that MBS is not part of mainstream medicine. However, the use of these principles has resulted in remarkable improvements in many patients' symptoms.

Resources for Stage III:

- *Unlearn Your Pain,* by Howard Schubiner, M.D.
- *The Art of Living* (modern interpretation of Epictetus by Sharon Lebell)

- Video *Cinema Paradiso* (short version)
- A support person to help you start looking upward and outward:
  - Life coach
  - Psychiatrist/psychologist
  - Religious leader
  - Healer

Checklist for Moving to Stage IV:

- Using "active meditation" throughout the day
- Consistently aware of the four different levels of awareness in your life: 1) environmental, 2) emotional, 3) judgment/"storytelling," and 4) ingrained patterns
- Read *Unlearn Your Pain* and took the test in Chapter 5 to see how MBS is affecting you
- Reading *The Art of Living* or another source of Epictetus's teachings regularly
- Watched *Cinema Paradiso*
- Aware of the devastating effects of "labeling." Identified and removed the labels you assigned to yourself and others.

This phase has no time frame—you'll be referring back to it frequently as you move forward.

Stage IV: Take Back Your Life

Many patients stop their journey at Stages II or III. It may be that they already feel so much better that they don't see the need to move forward. Their pain is usually gone or reduced to a level that's not interfering with their quality of life. But it's important to keep going: Stage IV helps you to consolidate your gains and integrate them into your life. It will set you up for long-lasting change.

Goals

Education

- Understand how much of your former life you have lost.
- Learn the tools that will help you regain it.

Sleep

- Should no longer be an issue
- Re-do prior sleep steps if a problem.

Central Nervous System

- Reconnect your nervous system to the best part of your life.
- Systematically establish the structure to create the best part of your life.
- Improve relationships with your family and friends.

Medications

- Begin to focus on getting off all medications.

Goal setting

- Main focus of Stage IV.
- Get organized.
- Develop "personal business plan."
- Make immediate family issues your highest priority.

Rehabilitation

- Continue with basic resistance training.
- Redevelop recreational activities that are physical.

Five Steps

Step 1: Connect with the Life You Desire

When you're in chronic pain life becomes very heavy. You develop a lifestyle based on merely surviving. You're just trying to keep your head above water as you deal with a significant amount of stress. Additionally, you're carrying a heavy pain burden. You may have forgotten what it's like to live your life with deep joy and excitement about the possibilities. I would suggest an exercise that I have personally found helpful.

First, find a quiet time and place where you can just think and possibly go into a meditative state. Think back to the time in your life when you were the happiest.

Next, visually take yourself back there, trying to remember every possible detail about that era of your life. Remember:

- Dreams/Goals
- Attitudes
- Friends
- Activities
- Feelings and emotions around specific events

Spend as much time as you can with this exercise and repeat it a few times. Later on in the process, you'll develop a plan for bringing joy back into your life, but don't worry about that now. Instead, just move on to Step 2.

Step 2: Implementing Your Vision—Three Questions

Here are exercises for putting three "vision" questions in writing, meant to jumpstart the thinking process and help you get organized.

Question #1: Where am I?

To answer this question, outline the important areas of your life. For each of these areas, assess in writing 1) your current situation and 2) the tools and resources you have to solve any problems.

- Health
  - General health
  - Chronic pain

- Family
- Friends
- Work/career
- Hobbies/Recreation

In thinking about your family life, consider how you fit into it. If you live with family members, imagine you are one of them seeing you walk in the door. Is your energy "happy, loving, and peaceful" or is it "angry and frustrated?" Would *you* want to live with you? Are you an inspiration to your spouse and children or are you taking out your frustrations on them?

Question #2: Where do I want to go?

After you've outlined and honestly assessed these aspects of your life, start developing your vision for each of them. You may feel you have a hundred reasons or excuses to not do this, but when will there be a better time? When is your life going to get easier so you can create your vision? Find a quiet place and take a half or full day to sit back and think about your life. Take a mental tour of all of it. Then recall the exercise in Step 1 where you remembered your life when you were the happiest.

Don't start developing your vision until you can regain the *feel* of what life was like when you were actively striving for your dreams. Be honest with yourself regarding all of this. Did you ever have dreams? Did you ever actively pursue them?

- Once you've recalled a joyous period of your life, sit down again and compare it to the present.
- Visualize the contrast between your current life and that happiest period.
- Note the gap between the periods.
- Make a commitment to pursue your dreams or passions.
- Write your vision in as much detail as you can. Try to stay connected to the feelings you experienced in Step 1. This is not a writing exercise that you throw away.

After you've taken time for the reflection, write down a life plan. Do it *without* taking your chronic pain into account. Think about how you'd like to live a fulfilling and enjoyable life in each of the areas from Question #1 (health, family, friends, work, hobbies).

Next do a vision for where you want to go in terms of dealing with your chronic pain. Take each area of the DOCC program and create a plan of action for each:

- Sleep
- Medication management
- Goal setting
- Education
- Stress
- Rehabilitation

Question #3: How do I get there?

Now combine the two visions together. Take your life vision and insert it into your vision for your chronic pain. After all, the two are intertwined. It's important to avoid thinking that if you could just get rid of the pain, your life could move forward. Instead, focus on the idea that you'll advance your life and the pain is going to do what it will do. The ultimate paradox is that by sequencing your thinking in this order, there's a much higher chance that your pain will ultimately become a non-issue.

Once the two visions are combined, make a master plan. Think about what you need to do to make your combined vision come to life. Use every tool you now have in your arsenal. Be honest and realistic.

Think of this as developing a personal "business plan." I've found this process personally very helpful. As discussed in Chapter 2, just assume that your life is a business and that there are certain short and long-term goals you'd like to achieve. As with any business start-up, you're more likely to succeed if you have a written plan, the more specific the better.

It may take a few months to get your plan implemented. It will also take a lot of effort and homework. But remember, this is your entire life at stake. What else do have to do that's more important than taking charge of your life and treating your chronic pain?

Share your goals with your doctor so that you can work together to reach them. Consider the steps you can take in each of the life areas of health, family, friends, work, and hobbies. Make them as detailed as you can.

Step 3: Get Organized

As I mentioned in Chapter 2, at one point in my life I was frustrated with my seeming inability to get stuff done. This included things that I really wanted to accomplish or experience. I was very disorganized. I've since learned that organizational skills are not inherent, they're learned. To step into the life you want to create, it's vital to have an organizational system. Here are some steps to take:

- Pick an organizational system you'd like to learn. (And don't just purchase a day planner.) There are many systems to choose from, and you'll need to learn the skills in order to take advantage of them. I've found David Allen's seminars and book, *Getting Things Done,*[7] invaluable.
- Decide whether you want to implement the system on paper or use a computer.
- Use the system you've chosen. Don't let yourself off the hook. It'll become much easier over time.
- Don't put anything on your "to do" list unless you intend to *do* it.

Step 4: Address Family Issues

Pain = frustration. With chronic pain the frustration is usually intense. When you're frustrated and angry, you're disconnected from what's immediately in front of you. Your awareness goes to zero, which leads to abusive behavior. You may think that you're aware, but your children undoubtedly see it much differently.

When you're angry, your kids—who are completely dependent on you—have no control and become fearful. At a minimum, you cease to be a source of peace, joy, and happiness within your family. It's likely you're not volunteering to be your kids' coach or taking an active role in their lives. However it's manifested, chronic pain takes a terrible toll on those close to you. Here are several suggestions for fostering healthy, loving interactions with family members that I've used successfully with my patients:

- Read the book *Parent Effectiveness Training*, by Thomas Gordon.[8] This classic has made the biggest impact on my life of any book I've read. It will increase your awareness of not only your children's needs but also those of your spouse or partner.
- Do not engage with your family if you are angry—EVER!!!! Do not re-engage until you are completely calm.
- Ask your family what it's like to be around you when you're upset.
  - Write their answers down and look at what you've written, or bring it to mind, whenever you're tempted to interact with any of them while you're angry.
- Listen to your children without giving advice or an opinion unless you're asked. (This action step is courtesy of Hyde School.)
  - I usually ask my patients to commit to doing this for a month to begin the process. It should evolve into a lifetime habit.
- Work with all members of your family to create a vision of what they'd like their family life to look like.
  - Institute a tradition of having a family meeting with an agenda once a week. (Hyde School again.)

You need your family for your support. Don't become a living weapon with them as your target.

Step 5: The Hoffman Process

There are many personal growth centers and programs across the country to choose from. The Hoffman Process is an eight-day in-house experience that has enhanced my own life immeasurably. Hoffman-trained teachers explain how to break up entrenched neurological pathways and reprogram your responses to the events that trigger them. In other words, instead of experiencing "stimulus, then response," the pattern becomes "stimulus, then *choice* of response." The tools this program offers help you learn how to break the compulsive link between any given situation and your automatic response. In my experience, reprogramming work which would take years on your own can be accomplished in these eight days.

There's a strong connection between the Hoffman techniques and the Mind Body Syndrome. The essence of MBS is that you have neurological pathways that will predictably become activated by a specific circumstance or level of stress. All of our responses to stress are essentially pre-programmed so that a specific stimulus will elicit a fairly predictable reaction. Any time you're anxious you're probably in a "pattern." Hoffman helps you to break out of the pattern.

Hoffman is not for everyone and it's also not within the budget of many people, but there are other programs and resources available that emphasize connecting thoughts with physical sensations. The term used to describe this type of process is "somatic work."

Resources for Stage IV:

- *Getting Things Done,* by David Allen
- *Parent Effectiveness Training,* by Thomas Gordon, M.D.
- Goal-setting tools in *Back in Control*
- Personal growth organizations

Checklist for Moving to Stage V:

- Visually and emotionally reconnected to who you were when you were the happiest
- Written a detailed personal "business plan"
- Learned and implemented an organizational system
- Read *Parent Effectiveness Training* and implemented many concepts
- Actively creating the family life that you desire
- Considered the Hoffman Process or a similar program/organization that uses somatic tools for change

STAGE V: LIVE LIFE TO THE FULLEST
Goals:

Education
- Review your whole experience

Sleep
- Restful full night's sleep with minimal sleep aids

Central Nervous System
- Establishing lifetime "maintenance" practices
- Embarking on your spiritual journey

Medications
- Off all pain, sleep, and anti-anxiety medications

Goal setting
- Reaching beyond yourself

Rehabilitation
- Aggressively pursuing all aspects of your health

Five Steps
Step 1: Understand the Importance
of Stepping into Your New Life

Probably the most powerful way of creating new neurological pathways is when you're engaged with your true value system and pursuing your interests based on that connection. I call this "living an engaged life."

Living an engaged life starts with gradually becoming more functional. This process unfolds as your focus shifts from your pain to becoming more active. Consider how your brain works: as discussed in Chapter 7, it's much like what happens on your drive home at the end of the day. As you drive, you see many things, but your brain won't remember every car, house, tree, and store that you pass; instead, you screen out most of it. This occurs because your nervous system is hierarchal. In other words, it remembers only what's most prominent. As you get further along in the healing process, your focus will be diverted from your pain onto your life—i.e., the pain circuits will move down the chain in terms of your attention. The enjoyable activities you do will start to "outrank" your pain. This is why rehabilitation physicians emphasize function over pain relief in their treatment of chronic pain. If you assume that you have to get rid of your pain before you can live your life, forget it. You're done. Your pain will progressively occupy more and more of your conscious thoughts.

Along these same lines, if you're engaging in activities only to distract yourself from your pain, you'll have the same problem. Your pain is still running the show. Do activities simply because you enjoy them and because they help you live a full and balanced life—don't hold on to any alternative agenda.

As discussed, part of becoming more functional is working on any anxiety and anger issues. When your thoughts and behavior aren't fueled by anxiety and anger, you can engage in your life with zeal. Keep in mind that it's not that you'll get rid of anxiety and frustration; it's that they will no longer control you. This frees you up to connect with yourself, family, friends, and the essence of your existence. At this point, adversity, including chronic pain, will not trump all else. New brain pathways will be created. It's astounding to me how much this approach has played a role in decreasing my patients' pain. I would never have predicted this sequence ten years ago.

Step 2: Establish Lifetime Practices—
The Power of Commitment

Commit to *scheduling* time daily or weekly to keep yourself using the strategies and tools you've found the most effective. With repetition, these more functional ways of living will become your baseline.

When I think of commitment, one particular event comes to mind. On Christmas Day, 2008, I went skiing with my son Nick and his friend Holt. One moment in the day found the three of us standing on top of a cornice at Snowbird, Utah. For you non-skiers, a cornice is a snow formation that occurs at the top of a mountain ridge. As the wind blows the snow up the mountain, a drop-off of ten to twenty feet is formed. Most skiers make a diagonal trail down this drop-off, which is fairly simple and safe. U.S. ski team skiers (like Nick as Holt) often jump straight off them.

Just below the cornice was a chute that was approximately twenty feet wide at the top but only about six feet wide two-thirds of the way down. About a hundred feet below us on the left there was an outcropping of rocks that stretched for two hundred feet.

Holt looked at it. "Holt," I said. "I don't think your coaches would be thrilled with the idea of you skiing down this." He looked at me and then immediately jumped into the chute. He skied about seventy-five feet straight down, made a gentle turn to the right, another gentle turn to the left and ended up in a large bowl. Nick skied to the right and jumped from a fifteen-foot cliff into the same chute, making the same turns. They were each traveling forty or fifty miles an hour when they reached the open bowl. This was simply an undoable chute for most human beings. It was clear that if they'd hesitated midway—if they hadn't remained committed to their decisions—they would've run the risk of serious injury.

Mind you, Nick's and Holt's certainty came from hours upon hours of practice over many years. They each knew they could make that jump because they're supremely confident skiers and had done tough jumps before. I hope you too can build this kind of certainty from practicing the skills that will propel you further along in your journey. Don't hesitate in your pursuit of your new life—commit to yourself and your new reality. Life is short.

Step 3: Your Journey Inward

It has been pointed out for centuries that the only person you can change in life is *you*. This is a very challenging concept for me in that from the time I decided to become a physician, my energy was focused on fixing people around me. In retrospect I realize that I was focused on others both to divert attention from myself and also to "save others to save myself."

Of course, I didn't perceive that I, personally, needed any work at all. Making this connection has been the most humbling part of my journey. Not only was I broken, I was really broken. It was under such severe stress that my façade crumbled.

The key to any success that I've had helping others with their problems has stemmed from me being more connected to myself. Connecting to myself has boosted my ability to simply talk to others human-to-human. My patients figure out how to heal themselves on their own. In fact, when they reconnect with who they are and where they want to go, there's no stopping them. It's similar to opening the door on a wild animal's cage. I've learned to just give advice when asked and stay out of the way. Every human, given a chance, wants to thrive.

There's a strong natural tendency among my patients as they begin to experience success with the "tools" discussed in this book to try to engage their family members in the process. Although I do strongly encourage both halves of a couple to engage, they each have to do it separately and of their own free will. Any energy focused by one on the other's progress is counter-productive.

Focusing on your own journey has an infinite number of elements. A few overall guidelines for you:

- Become aware of any energy you spend on trying to "fix" those around you. Instead, truly commit to your own growth.
- Develop an awareness of your own flaws and then learn to embrace and accept them. It's the first step in moving forward.
- Read an excerpt from *The Art of Living,* the teachings of Epictetus as interpreted by Sharon Lebell. His focus is almost completely on the journey inward.
- Carefully research and choose tools that will allow you to progress down this road.

Step 4: Your Spiritual Journey

My definition of a spiritual journey is quite broad. I define it as simply looking at and experiencing life outside of your own self. You're in the process of gaining (or regaining) a larger perspective that will lead you to lose your sense of self-importance and increase your awareness of others' needs. This requires conscious effort. There are an infinite number of ways to develop your spiritual life, but here are a few things to consider engaging in:

- Quality time with family and friends
- Spiritual organizations
- Good food, wines, etc.
- Energizing experiences
- Creative hobbies
- The arts

Any experience that involves active engagement and broadening your perspective works. This is particularly true when you can share it with others. Passive experiences such as watching TV are fine for relaxation, but, needless to say, they won't help you achieve spiritual growth.

Imagine what form your journey might take and *write it down*. Then review what you've written every six months or at least once a year.

Step 5: Giving Back

The final step of the twenty-five in this chapter is giving back. The urge to give back grows out of empathy, which is an inherent part of the human experience. Empathy is the ability to see a situation through another person's eyes with an understanding of what it might be like to be in a similar circumstance. It's often accompanied by a desire to help out.

From an evolutionary perspective, the group of humans who learned to cooperate had the highest likelihood of survival. The reason that many people seem so self-centered and self-serving is, paradoxically, that they've been disconnected from them-*selves* by anxiety and anger. It's not possible to reach out to others if you're just trying to survive emotionally.

Once you've implemented the tools that will reconnect you to your "authentic self" (Hoffman) you'll have the desire, energy, and ability to reach out to others. I've observed this happening in my patients and it has been my personal experience as well.

Patients free of pain want to give back—and in a big way. I have a patient who was left paraplegic from an unfortunate series of events surrounding spine surgery. Reading and using the book *Forgive for Good* made a tremendous impact on her outlook, mood, and pain. After she embraced true forgiveness, her overwhelming urge was to help others in wheelchairs who were suffering from chronic pain. She's now happier in a wheelchair than she was walking, anxious and angry.

I have a few suggestions that might help you formulate your own ideas about how to give back:

- Stay committed to your own journey.
- Remain aware of the fact that aside from yourself, your highest priority is your immediate family.
- Read Karen Armstrong's book *Twelve Steps to a Compassionate Life.*[9] She is an international religious leader who in this book outlines the history of compassion and highlights the importance of nurturing and practicing it.
- Make a random list of ideas about giving back that are interesting to you. Then:
  - Pick the top five.
  - Prioritize them.
  - Develop a specific plan of how you are going to make it happen. Do it!!

Resources for Stage V:

- *Twelve Steps to Live a Compassionate Life,* by Karen Armstrong
- *The Art of Living,* by Sharon Lebell (Epictetus)
- Outside help such as organizations, healers, psychologists, psychiatrists, seminars, church, etc.

Living in Stage V:

We are what we repeatedly do.
Excellence, then, is not an act, but a habit.

—Aristotle

MISCELLANEOUS HOMEWORK
Active Self-Discovery

There are an infinite number of resources that provide tools to help you live a more satisfying life. In this chapter I've listed just a few. In looking back, I think that everything I tried or read added something to help me in my own journey. The problem I had was that whenever I found a new tool, I'd feel that it was the complete solution to all my problems and the key to transforming my life.

I feel strongly that I wouldn't have been on an endless search to "fix" myself if I'd been taught stress management skills in middle or high school. If I'd had the skills, I could've processed stress in a more constructive way. Instead of having the knowledge I needed to live a full interactive life, I was always in survival mode.

In retrospect, it seems incredible to me that I was put through the rigors of fifteen years of medical training AFTER high school without a clue about how to effectively deal with stress. And the training part was easy in comparison to the stresses of private practice. Somehow I ended up choosing one of the most taxing careers within medicine. I feel fortunate to have made it through somewhat intact.

I would encourage you to actively pursue every avenue available to improve your ability to process stress. You'll connect with some and not others. All of it will be uncomfortable and some of it painful, but it will enable you to live a better, more satisfying life.

I now feel that not only do I have a responsibility to myself to grow, but I have a responsibility to model better ways of behaving. I don't want to pass along my family of origin's pathology to my own children. I don't want to treat my wife the same way my parents treated each other.

Psychotherapy/Counseling

At one point in my life I thought that traditional psychological counseling was the only way to deal with stress. Then I became focused on cognitive behavioral therapy as the best method. The reality is that many techniques and schools of thought can be helpful. Many situations we find ourselves in are complicated and require extra insight to handle. Whenever possible, obtain the help of a therapist. A therapist can shed light on your specific issue. Moral support is also critical.

For some reason, many people are resistant to seeking psychotherapy. I am always perplexed as to why that would be the case. We all have experienced less than perfect modeling from our parents. I have yet to meet anyone from a perfectly "functional" family that has left them with no emotional baggage. I think of life as a backpacking trip. Why would you go on the trip with fifty pounds of rocks in your pack in addition to basic supplies? Therapy helps you unload those useless rocks.

I would suggest that if you don't believe in therapy—or just plain don't want to go—you're choosing to remain a victim of your circumstances. Why would you, instead, want me to perform an operation on you that carries significant risk and has an unpredictable chance of success? Tell me, exactly, what is the downside risk of talking to a therapist?

Self-Help Books

There are tens of thousands of self-help books available. During one period of my life I was obsessive about reading one after another. I do feel that they can be a helpful and even necessary piece of working on oneself. They represent a "didactic" phase of learning about life skills and most are written by smart, experienced people.

Finally, however, my counselor ordered me to quit reading these books. He saw the danger they posed, which is that they can become a substitute for actual change. I tended to intellectualize them and they became another part of my identity. Although I thought I'd made the correct changes, I hadn't gone into the experiential phase enough to have anything really take place; it was all conceptual. However, they did sow the seeds for real change.

Structured Seminars

Attending structured seminars focused on self-discovery can be a good step toward finding your true self because they add an experiential level to the process. In addition, sharing what you're learning with others who are on the same quest is very powerful.

There are many seminars available. I don't have any specific recommendations; I think most of them have a lot of potential value if you commit to the process and can "connect" to it. If, by chance, you have negative feelings about a given seminar, it might be because you have different needs, or because you're not ready to deal with the issues it has raised, or maybe because seminars are simply not an effective resource for you. Just don't give up on the self-discovery process as a whole.

My family and I have benefitted greatly from the structured seminars that my stepdaughter's boarding school, Hyde, sponsors three times a year. She was a student there for her junior and senior years of high school. This was during a period when our family was struggling mightily with her transition into adulthood. The school's philosophy is based on the premise that knowledge in and of itself does not prepare you adequately for a successful life; they focus first and foremost on the student's character. They set up the seminars because much of everyone's character is shaped by his or her interaction with family. It was a unique experience in that prior to this experience I had not really bonded with my stepdaughter. These family seminars included my wife, her ex-husband, and myself. Once a year it was just my stepdaughter and me.

I was initially quite cynical about the whole idea. I'd already done a lot of work on myself and wasn't sure what else I could learn. In these group sessions, I would often spend a lot of time and effort "sharing my wisdom." I had learned a lot and did have a lot to offer. However, as others pointed out, "it's difficult to learn with your mouth open."

In January of 2007, I was attending a one-on-one weekend. The week before, my regional west coast Hyde group had worked me over about issues with my son that I hadn't seen very clearly. I was not in a great mood. I was a little negative and had decided to not contribute much to the group. What I didn't realize was that as a result I would end up actually listening.

I watched one father try to be the perfect Hyde seminar parent. He was a great, well-intentioned guy, but these very qualities were clearly blocking him from connecting with his son. I realized how often I had played that role in my own life.

One of the exercises was to write a final letter to myself about my core values. I decided to open up my mind a little more and asked myself the question, "If I'm so enlightened, why am I such a workaholic?" During the seminar, a story kept popping into my head from when I was a first-year resident in orthopedics at Queen's Hospital in Honolulu, Hawaii. About three months into my training I overheard one of the other residents talking about admitting a patient with severe back pain who also had a significant anxiety disorder. I asked him, "What do you mean by anxiety disorder?" I had no idea what anxiety was; I had to look it up in a textbook.

Eventually I developed a severe anxiety disorder myself. As I sat in the Hyde seminar room looking back, I couldn't figure out how I could have gone through college, medical school, and two years of internal medicine residency and not have had a clue about the nature of anxiety. Obviously I'd encountered many anxiety-provoking situations.

That afternoon a bomb went off in my head. Anxiety, in fact, was all that I knew. I'd been raised in an abusive household, never knowing when my mother would explode. She was, at some level, experiencing rage most of the time. Because of this, fear was the basis of all of my behavior going forward. Most of my energy as a child was spent trying not to set my mother off and/or calming her down. Most of my energy in adulthood was spent in avoiding unpleasant emotions: I dealt with anger by suppressing it and I addressed anxiety by staying distracted, mostly by my work.

Hyde set up the structure for me to have these realizations. The didactic part of it was critical, but my paradigm shift would not have occurred without the support of the people in that room. They were part of something that permanently changed my life.

HOMEWORK SUMMARY

I've just suggested a sequence of homework. Note that there's a specific reason I suggest going through it in this order.

First of all, it's important to learn as much as possible about the variables that affect your perception of pain. Then start working on your anxiety. Anxiety has to be dealt with before anger for two reasons. As discussed, anger effectively covers up the feeling of anxiety. If you address anger first, you're exposed to raw anxiety without adequate tools to cope. Secondly, anxiety is a significant reason that many people in chronic pain don't sleep well. Without sleep none of this process is effective.

Anger is addressed next because it keeps the anxiety and pain circuits fired up. I have consistently observed patients who work through their anger become pain-free.

Often people stop after Stage II, as they are feeling so much better; frequently even better than before the chronic pain began. So why go any further? What people don't grasp is that they have just begun the journey. The goal is to experience a massive shift in consciousness, one that not only makes your pain a distant bad memory, but also allows you to create a life that you never thought possible.

Stage III introduces you to a whole different set of tools and concepts that you can use to expand your consciousness. The writing tools are critical; there's no substitute for free writing and the Feeling Good exercises. However, they will only carry you so far. Becoming more aware and skilled at recognizing all four levels of awareness will dramatically enhance your quality of life. This includes making active meditation a basic part of each day.

Stage IV is designed to help you consolidate the gains you've made and get organized before you engage in the final leg of this journey.

Stage V is what this whole book is about. Your brain/mind has now healed itself and can live in a different place than it did when dominated by chronic pain. If you engage in tools that allow you to expand your life, you'll find that the topic of pain becomes very uninteresting and the pain circuits will be weakened.

It's important to use the set of tools that are best suited for you on a regular basis. Otherwise you'll quickly slip back into your set patterns of behavior. Refer back to this chapter as an ongoing reference. You can also check www.back-in-control.com.

The DOCC Project is a work in progress and so are you. Welcome to your new life. Enjoy it!!

CHAPTER 10
Excellent Rehabilitation

O ver time, I've come to learn in my practice that it's pointless to engage a patient in aggressive rehab until his or her nervous system has been calmed down. It doesn't have to be entirely calmed down, but he or she must be actively engaged in using stress management tools with some noticeable benefit. Reading this book up to this chapter is a good start. I would also urge you to fully engage in the homework from Chapter 9 or in other stress reduction techniques that fit with your learning style and outlook.

To address the soft tissues with manual physical therapy, they must be vigorously manipulated. Invariably, this manipulation causes some degree of pain, sometimes a high degree. At whatever level, a patient in chronic pain will feel it even more acutely: recall the experiment cited in Chapter 1, where a functional MRI scan revealed that the brain's response to a pain impulse markedly increases after more than twelve months of being in pain. If the added pain from the physical therapy is too much for you to cope with, you may become frustrated and step back onto the down escalator.

Effective rehabilitation also requires active, motivated physical participation. I'm always slightly amused at the gym when I see someone on a stationary bicycle with the pedals barely moving. That's not exercising. While it's okay to start slow if you haven't worked out in a while, your effort needs to increase with each gym visit in order to produce any significant benefit. Just showing up won't help you get in shape.

As with any profession, the skill level and training among different physical therapists varies greatly—that's why it's important to assess your own therapy. If you're fortunate enough to work with a great therapist the first time around, terrific. But if you aren't, don't hesitate to switch.

I have no personal expertise in physical therapy; I can only tell you some of what I've learned to expect from the practitioners I work with. I'm fortunate in that Seattle has a remarkable standard of physical therapy—the vast majority of therapists here have a base of knowledge that far exceeds the requirement for treating spinal disorders. Most have taken advanced training in manual therapy. This excellence may stem from the fact that historically physiatrists in the area have demanded a high quality of therapy; I noticed it when I first started practice twenty-five years ago. The culture continues to carry on that tradition.

I choose to work with just a few therapists regularly, as I like to be able to communicate quickly with them about my patients' status. They also know exactly what I expect. I frequently quiz my patients about their physical therapy experience. If a patient is coming to see me from out of town, I'll often get in contact with their local therapist to explain the patient's problem and let them know my expectations. I also want to make sure that they have a certain degree of expertise in spine therapy.

There are several components I feel are necessary for superior physical therapy:

- Education
  - Anatomy
  - Function
  - Awareness of harmful activities
  - Strategies to be safely functional

- Assessment
  - Spine mechanics
  - Muscle imbalances around the spine
  - Postural issues
- Advanced soft tissue skills
  - Assessment of each motion segment of your spine, including increased vs. decreased mobility
  - Identification of painful segments
- Long-term home conditioning program
  - Core stabilization
  - Flexibility
  - Generalized conditioning

It's beyond the scope of this chapter to cover the above-mentioned variables in detail. My goal is to give you enough information so you can evaluate the quality of therapy you are receiving.

GENERAL CONCEPTS
Demand the Best

There's a chance you just read the list of components above and thought, "I didn't go through all that when *I* got physical therapy." And most likely you also didn't get better. Although a lot of therapists in my area do cover all of these bases, there are also many that don't. When I have a patient with ongoing low back pain, I always ask what kind of therapy they've already had. Frequently I discover that it's been limited to some ultrasound, heat, ice, and/or light massage. Vital aspects of the process have been overlooked, such as an evaluation of pelvic girdle muscle balance or a discussion of any workplace or lifestyle demands on the back. I'll find out that education wasn't done, and that there's no long-term plan in place.

So the first step if a patient in my care has had unsatisfactory therapy is to send them to a therapy group that *does* cover all the bases. I would estimate that over half the time, that step alone solves the problem.

So why am I so wired about demanding a certain level of training and expertise when it comes to physical therapy? Think about this for a minute. The quality of your physical therapy plays a huge role in your recovery from chronic back pain. Many patients who've had inadequate physical therapy services conclude that therapy has "failed" when, in fact, they haven't really given it a fair chance. They become frustrated at the lack of improvement and opt for surgery when it may be unnecessary. The most common reason given for performing a spine fusion or inserting an artificial disc to relieve low back pain is "failure of conservative care."

Adequate conservative care is the focus of this whole book. At a minimum, you should have worked hard on rehabilitation for at least six months before surgery even enters your mind. These operations are major and they don't work that well. You must take full responsibility to see that you're receiving thorough, effective physical therapy. All of this is a high stakes game.

A lot of my patients tell me they don't have time to pursue aggressive rehabilitation. Really? The pain you're suffering is affecting and enveloping *every* aspect of your life. Remember, not fully pursuing a treatment that would significantly improve your quality of life is one of the most common ways of remaining in victim mode.

I am fifty-nine years old at this moment and have a heavy workload: I often work fifty to seventy hours a week. I'm not necessarily proud of that anymore, and I'm trying to tone it all down, yet I still have surgical days that are ten to fourteen hours long, sometimes for just one case. If I didn't get to the gym for three to five hours a week every week, I wouldn't have the strength and endurance to do my job.

Desensitizing the Soft Tissues

When the nervous system is subjected to a chronic, repetitive stimulus, it becomes overly responsive. All the healing elements we've covered so far—improving sleep, dealing with anxiety and anger in a proactive way, cognitive behavioral theory, improving function, and substituting new circuit patterns for old—contribute to the desensitization process. The other crucial piece of this process is to work directly on the soft tissues.

Consider the cycle of pain that occurs when the soft tissues are injured. First, there's the injury, which, when it occurs in the low back, is often dramatic and severe. The initial pain causes anxiety. Then the anxiety causes you to guard the painful area (i.e., not use it), thereby making the tissues stiff. Movement exacerbates the pain and leads to more guarding, especially if the tissue is moved too quickly or with too much force. As the brain starts to focus on the pain, the pain circuits intensify, which again leads to more guarding and stiffness. Guarding typically lasts a few weeks and then resolves. If it continues for several months, however, the soft tissues won't move as easily or as well.

My patients find it difficult to understand that the pain can get worse without additional injury; guarding—an act people think protects their back—is actually one of the contributing factors. All soft tissue is protected by pain-inducing fibers that are stimulated when the physical limit of that tissue is reached. For example, take your wrist and bend it forward with your other hand as far as you can. What happens when you reach the limit of your flexion? It hurts. If you then try to push it further, it hurts a lot. Now imagine your wrist being in a cast for six weeks. Anyone who's lived with a cast knows that the worst part is taking it off because the joint is stiff and sore. If you were to repeat the wrist-bending experiment at this point, you'd only have to move it a third to half as much to produce the *same* pain response.

Physical therapists work to resolve pain by pushing the limits of the contracted soft tissues to allow a full range of motion before the patient feels pain. The stretching increases the tissue's flexibility, which then allows more motion. The therapists take into account that the nervous system is overly sensitive, and so try to keep the pain caused by therapy at a tolerable level. Gradually, with repetitive stretching and controlled stimulation of the nervous system, the pain will diminish.

THE BASIC COMPONENTS
Education

To get the most out of your physical therapy, it's critical to become fully aware of *all* aspects of your spine care. A given round of physical therapy may solve a specific episode of back pain, but understanding the full context of your problem will keep you from reinjuring the tissue.

Your education should include an overview of spinal anatomy provided by either your therapist, a book, a website, or all three. The more visual the process, the better. By becoming comfortable with the basic language, you can communicate with your health care providers more clearly.

The second step is to understand how specific movements such as bending and lifting improperly can potentially strain and injure the soft tissues that support your spine and the discs inside your vertebrae. It's important to be as specific as possible with your therapist about what aspects of your lifestyle are potentially irritating to your spine. By working with your therapist and learning how your back functions, you can develop new patterns that help you to avoid injury. This is much more effective than trying to memorize a list of what you can and cannot do. If you don't know what you're doing to irritate your back, how are you going to correct it?

There's more to the education process: as discussed, part of it is learning that in many cases there's no structural source of your pain that can be "fixed" with surgery. This realization can be extremely frustrating for patients. Just because there's no quick fix, though, doesn't mean that the pain isn't there. And the pain can be reduced if you take steps such as engaging in a conditioning program. In their frustration patients often don't want to commit to working out; they want the easy way out, looking to outside sources to "cure" them. Thinking like this, however, is a very passive way of caring for your health. It's not dissimilar to being markedly overweight and bemoaning your knee arthritis, hypertension, and diabetes. If you choose to remain passive about your health, that's fine, but you do lose your right to complain about it. You also cannot expect the medical profession to make up for a completely self-inflicted set of diseases.

There are other concepts to become familiar with: as we talked about in Chapter 1, it's possible that you have a soft tissue injury that's not showing up on an MRI. Consider that if you sprained your knee, that wouldn't show up on an MRI either. You could keep re-spraining it and it *still* wouldn't show up, and yet you'd still be in pain.

Even if you have no specific diagnosis, know that the body's pain system is designed to fire when excessive force is applied to a normal tissue. That's why the entire system exists—it's incredibly well designed. If the tissues are already damaged or inflamed, even less outside force will stimulate the pain circuits.

The Mind Body Syndrome is the most difficult pain-related concept to understand, but it may be the most common source of ongoing pain. Once your pain pathways are established they are permanently embedded in your brain. Stress can cause them to become reactivated at any time. My veteran patients are very aware of this link.

If you haven't learned about and *incorporated* the above concepts into your approach to healing, you haven't even started rehab. Why would you want to undergo a major spine surgery or continue to suffer severe pain without first addressing the basics?

Basic Spine Care

Although many therapists cover a lot of material during a physical therapy session, it's not the right setting in which to get a full overview. They may not have time to cover all the details, and a typical, active physical therapy session is filled with distractions. That's why it's a good idea to look to other resources to learn basic spine care concepts.

At our hospital we have a program called "Back on Track" that helps patients become more informed about the rehab process. Groups of eight to twelve people meet in two sessions of two hours each to discuss different strategies for dealing with daily activities, and the activities are demonstrated and then practiced by the group. The goal is to learn by listening, doing, and asking questions, and there's also a lot of sharing. Regardless of where my patients are receiving their physical therapy, I ask them to attend these classes; while much of the information may already be known, the classes help fill in the gaps. The feedback has been uniformly positive. I recently had one long-term back pain patient markedly decrease her pain by changing just one activity she'd been doing improperly.

If you don't have access to this type of resource, there are an abundant number of websites and books that can be effective in teaching you about spine care.

If you've experienced back pain for an extended period of time, have you taken the time to look up and learn as much as you can about the anatomy and function of your spine? If not, why not? Again, not doing so is one way of remaining a victim. The information you need is widely available.

Urban Legends

Another part of the educational process is learning what's *not* the source of your chronic pain. There are many urban legends out there that are frightening to patients with back pain. This is especially true if the pain has become chronic.

One common scenario is when patients are told they have an ailment called degenerative disc disease. Allow me to clear up the confusion right now: this is not a disease! I recall one sixty-year-old gentleman I saw many years ago who'd been experiencing back pain for about eight weeks. He was terrified because he'd been told he had degenerated discs. He feared paralysis and loss of function. I explained to him in detail that his spine was *completely* normal for his age. All of his discs *had* degenerated, but discs normally degenerate with age. As I pointed out earlier in the book, there is no correlation between degenerated discs and back pain. Armed with that information, the man's anxiety lessened and his pain immediately diminished a significant amount. It's common, if the not the rule, that just knowing the problem isn't serious will decrease your perception of pain.

Assessment

On your first visit to physical therapy, your therapist should perform an extensive assessment of these factors:

- Posture
- Flexibility of your spine
- Tenderness of the soft tissues
- Flexibility of your hips, knees, and ankles
- Your pain tolerance

Your therapist may treat only your lower back symptoms for a given acute episode, but this is the wrong approach. Often there's a soft tissue imbalance that needs to be addressed to prevent the symptoms from coming back.

I'll give you a few examples. A common problem that occurs with aging is that as your discs degenerate you lose the curvature of your lower back. The normal curvature is referred to as "lordosis." This lordosis allows your head to stay centered over your pelvis, which minimizes the forces needed to stay balanced. As you lose this curvature, there's a tendency to feel like you're tipping forward. The term we use for this situation is "flatback." You can compensate for this imbalance in several ways. If you walk with your knees slightly bent, it will allow you to be more upright. However, your quads may quickly tire and the muscles in your lower back and buttock area will be forced to fire much more than usual. With time, the tissues in your groin will shorten and it will become even more difficult to stand upright without pain. A thorough assessment would check out all of these variables, and the treatment would include stretching out the hips, mobilizing the spine segments to improve curvature, and calming down the inflamed tissues. If only the lower back was addressed, your symptoms would be recurrent and persistent.

Another issue occurs when a large band of tissue that runs down the sides of both your legs, called the iliotibial (IT) band, becomes inflamed. This band, which connects the pelvis to the lower leg, is critical for balance and function. When it's inflamed, the pain can be severe. The pain path matches the one from the fifth lumbar nerve root, so it's possible to mistake this tendonitis in the IT band for sciatica. Therapists with excellent soft tissue skills can usually tell the difference. Just pushing on this band and assessing the tightness (instead of assuming it's sciatica based on the symptoms) will reveal tendonitis, which can be treated effectively in therapy, allowing you to avoid having to get an MRI scan of your back.

I recall a situation early in my practice where I had evaluated a patient for low back pain; it was a soft tissue problem and I prescribed physical therapy. On his return visit I noted that a lot of his pain was in his iliotibial band. I called up the therapist and asked why they hadn't treated the IT band tendonitis. The answer was, "You only wrote a prescription for us to treat the lower back." That was the last time I used that particular therapist.

Hip arthritis is commonly experienced as pain down the front of your thigh when walking. It's also the pain pathway for the fourth lumbar nerve root. At least twice a year I discover that a patient sent to me for sciatica actually has hip arthritis. Putting the hips through a range of motion quickly reveals the correct diagnosis. One patient I ran across many years ago had undergone four failed spine surgeries when the problem all along was hip arthritis.

A final example: I have seen several patients treated for a pulled hamstring when the problem was a ruptured L5-S1 disc. The misdiagnosis occurs because the first sacral nerve root (S1) travels down the area of the hamstrings. Simply palpating the hamstrings would have clarified the diagnosis.

It's not your responsibility to figure out these diagnoses or pinpoint other factors that may affect your treatment and outcome; it's the job of your physician and therapist. I've included these examples to increase your awareness of what should be done to obtain an accurate diagnosis. If you feel you've only had minimal assessment from your health care providers, then talk to your physician. If he or she seems unconcerned, find another doctor.

Advanced Soft Tissue Work

Advanced tissue work in the form of manual physical therapy can be extremely effective for patients with chronic pain. Part of your assessment process should include finding out your therapist's level of skill in this area. You can do so by asking what kind of training they've had—it should be extensive. More importantly, you can assess their skills by how aggressively you are physically being treated. If the treatment is passive, chances are they don't have advanced skills. I have an advantage in that I routinely ask my patients what types of treatment their physical therapists are utilizing.

When I first moved to Seattle in 1986, my physiatrist friend, Stan Herring, had me spend some time with a couple of excellent manual therapists, John Miller and his wife, Sue, whom he had recruited to Seattle. It was around this time that most of the therapists in the Seattle area really increased their level of spine care training, especially in the area of manual therapy.

I thought I'd be able to pick up a few pointers from John and Sue in terms of how to better examine my patients in my office. I quickly learned, however, that it was impossible for me to duplicate the sensitivity they had developed in their hands after examining thousands of patients. It's an important skill, one that requires both training and experience to develop. I felt that manual therapy had some similarities to surgery in that regard.

With complete deference to the manual therapy experts, I have a simplistic concept of what they do, divided into two categories:

- Segmental mobilization
- Myofascial work
    - Directly around the spine
    - Surrounding soft tissues and joints

One vertebral segment is defined as two vertebrae and the disc in between. Most patients have five "motion segments," i.e., segments that move. A few people have four or six. A good manual therapist can assess by feel how much a segment moves compared to the next one. The goal is to have all the segments move about the same amount. Therapists can also determine by feel and movement which segment is painful.

In examining segment movement, there are many possible combinations to be discovered. For example, four of the five segments might be stiff while the fifth moves too much, which implies that the more mobile segment is absorbing too much force. With repetition throughout the day, this hyper-mobile segment could become irritated, and so the idea would be to increase the motion of the other segments by manually manipulating them. You would then have a more even distribution of forces throughout all of the lumbar motion segments.

Another common situation is that all of the segments in the lower back are stiff. To my mind the solution to this issue is a little more debatable. If the whole spine is stiff and the actual segments aren't moving much, then the spine is less likely to be the source of pain. (Also note that mobilizing all of the spinal motion segments requires a significant commitment of time and is typically very painful.) It's more likely that the pain comes from the supporting soft tissues around the spine. In this case, it's my feeling that you should try to increase the mobility of the soft tissues around the hips to allow more motion there, causing less motion and stress across the back. Even when I perform a fusion of the entire spine from the neck to the pelvis, there's still some flexibility left; patients can still bend forward at the hips. I realize this is my own view—and arguable—but I have seen improved hip mobility decrease back pain many times.

Next comes myofascial work. Myofascial is a term that refers to the combination of a given muscle and the thin, tough layer of tissue that envelopes it, called "fascia." Muscles themselves do not contain pain fibers; it's the fasciae that contain an abundant number of them. The fascia is the layer that may become inflamed and very painful.

As described above, with pain there's an instinctive tendency to guard the injured area. As a result of chronic limitation of motion, the tissues will shorten. When you then try to put them through a normal range of motion, they will be painful and remain irritated.

Myofascial work is focused on specific massage techniques to identify which structures are inflamed and shortened and then stretch them out. As you might imagine, if you take an inflamed shortened muscle and perform a directed deep massage, it can be a painful process. The pain can be decreased somewhat with ice, ultrasound, and some of the other modalities of physical therapy. Good myofascial work is going to be painful, however; there's no way around it.

In an example above I mentioned the idea of improving hip movement, which is necessary for any thorough back treatment. Manual therapy includes stretching out the hip capsule with large motions and also working on specific tight myofascial structures around the hip.

Practitioners spend years learning and perfecting these soft tissue techniques. I've provided just a few simple examples to give you a feel for the concept. It's remarkable to me how an excellent manual therapist can improve flexibility and decrease soft tissue pain.

Most chiropractors have expertise in mobilization and soft tissue techniques. They are also allowed to perform "manipulations," where a higher force is used to put a given joint through a wider range of motion. They offer a wide range of methods. I have worked with many chiropractors who have greatly helped my patients in dealing with non-specific low back pain.

Whether a therapist or a chiropractor performs the soft tissue work, it's critical to combine it with the key components of education, assessment, and a long-term plan.

Long-Term Conditioning

If you've read this much of this book, you've probably experienced more low back pain than you would like. To gain any short or long-term relief, physical fitness is crucial.

The first part of any conditioning plan is to incorporate what you've learned about posture and body mechanics into your daily activities. It's the most important step, taken to avoid re-irritating tissues that you've finally persuaded to calm down. No amount of fitness will over-ride continuing to place abnormal stresses across the painful area.

As you address body mechanics, note that the spine is not well designed for upright posture. Your upper and lower body are connected by just this one structure (your spine) that is inherently unstable. Without the support of your trunk muscles and the small muscles directly connected to the spinal column, the spine would buckle and collapse with only four pounds of force applied to it.[1] Trunk support consists of: 1) the abdominal muscles, 2) the abdominal contents, which are liquid and provide support (similar to the bladder inside of a basketball), and 3) the surrounding muscle groups.[2]

It's often thought that if you lose weight, your low back pain will resolve. I have, in fact, observed the opposite phenomenon. As my patients have lost weight, their back pain often gets worse. This is likely because there's less tissue within the abdominal cavity for the muscles to compress against, and therefore less support. Don't get me wrong—I strongly favor losing weight. However, your priority should first be general conditioning and developing muscle tone. The weight will gradually come off. Once you're more physically fit, any lost weight will be less likely to cause an increase in low back pain.

I have a mantra I repeat to my patients over and over again: "I want you working out in the gym three to five hours per week the rest of your life." Many people just roll their eyes. You can choose not to work out, but know that it will be difficult if not impossible to recover from your pain if you're out of shape.

It's been shown that people over forty-five receive a tremendous benefit from weight training. We all lose a certain percentage of muscle mass every year (estimated to be about one percent), so resistance training becomes more important as we age. With weight training, you not only prevent the loss, you can also significantly improve your strength.

I prefer weight training to be done outside of the patient's home. There's something about having weights in the basement that just doesn't lend itself to frequent use. I think it's critical to get into an environment where others are working out hard as well; in addition, the equipment is much better.

Pilates is also excellent in that it emphasizes core strength, and I think yoga can be helpful if the extreme postures across the lower back are avoided.

I have a running argument with my therapists about the need for core training vs. gross weight training. Core exercises emphasize posture and focus on the small muscles next to the spine. The therapists feel that weight training doesn't train the core muscles enough to be effective for healing/preventing back pain. I do agree that working on the core muscles is critical in the acute and sub-acute phase of your back pain. However, in my experience—including being a back pain sufferer myself—it's not humanly possible to sustain doing these exercises over a long period of time; they're too boring. Good general core awareness and adherence to proper body mechanics plus conditioning with weights in the gym will maintain your spine health for a long time.

SUMMARY OF EXCELLENT REHABILITATION

It's estimated that only about 15% of Americans exercise on a regular basis.[3] I'm not sure why this number is so low—I personally want to be able to do what I've always done physically. I don't want to be limited.

I am an expert snow skier, but I don't come close to my son Nick and his best friend Holt. Anyone with a racing background will destroy me. I am able, though, to ski with Nick on almost any slope. He has become nice enough to do a lot of waiting. At fifty-nine, it would just not be possible to experience some of the best times of my life without being somewhat disciplined about staying in shape.

My father-in-law, who passed away at age ninety, started a vigorous twice-a-week gym program at around age seventy-five. When I asked him why he started his new regime, he said that he simply wanted to add fifteen yards to his drive on the golf course. He also just wanted to be able to play golf with his son. As a result of this commitment, he lived a normal physical life with few limitations. He played tennis twice a week and could hit a golf ball about a hundred and seventy-five yards up to six months before he became ill. Why wouldn't you want to remain fully physically functional for as long as possible?

Aside from remaining physically fit for its own sake, consider that you're experiencing pain that's destroying your quality of life. If you're contemplating surgery, also think about the fact that spine surgery is unpredictable in resolving low back pain. You may be in the cycle of not exercising because of your chronic pain and becoming less physically fit. Being in bad physical shape leads to even more pain. That cycle is deadly.

I've spent a large portion of this book discussing how to calm down your nervous system. One benefit of calming your nervous system by handling stress in a proactive way is that you have more mental energy to commit to exercising. Actively engaging in a conditioning program takes not only a substantial commitment of time but also strength of mind. In addition, a calmer nervous system helps you cope with the increased pain you'll experience during the initial phases of physical therapy.

Many factors affect your perception of pain. Your physical conditioning and flexibility is a major one. Insist on all four areas of rehab being covered:

- Education
- Thorough assessment

- Advanced soft tissue work
- Long-term conditioning program

Become an active participant in asking the right questions and setting up your own rehabilitation plan. Your quality of life depends on it.

CHAPTER 11

Do You Really Need Surgery?

Many people are skeptical about spine surgery, especially if they have a friend, neighbor, colleague, or family member who has undergone multiple surgeries and ended up with a deformity or ongoing pain. Unfortunately this poor reputation is deserved. Spine surgery performed for vague reasons often ends up with bad results. However, if done right, surgery can also be seemingly miraculous. To decide whether surgery is the best option for you, you should be aware of everything that influences the outcome. For example, it's important to know if your non operative care has been extensive enough—and good enough— for you to conclude that nothing else can be done. You can and should know exactly where you fit into the spectrum.

My goal here is to provide you with enough information so you can make a better shared decision with your doctor about surgery. But remember, in the end the decision to get surgery is yours alone—your surgeon is only making a recommendation.

Failure of Non-Operative Care?

Back in the fall of 2005, I attended a national spine meeting in Philadelphia. I was with one of my partners who is also a spine surgeon. We'd just heard two papers regarding the results of lumbar fusions in patients who were injured on the job and were on worker's compensation. The results were not very good; in fact, they were just slightly better than having no surgery at all. The main reason cited for performing the fusions in the first place was "failure of conservative care." ("Conservative care" is another term for "non-operative" care.) As my partner and I discussed the presentation, it occurred to us the speaker hadn't included a definition of "failed conservative care." And we realized that although we'd heard that term for all of our careers, a generally agreed-upon standard did not exist. This chapter will discuss the current state of affairs for deciding whether to perform a fusion for low back pain and suggest a possible definition of conservative care. The rough consensus among many physicians is that non-operative care is adequate if the patient has been treated for three to six months, including:

- Six to twelve physical therapy visits
- One to three cortisone injections
- An evaluation by a psychologist who specializes in dealing with pain, which is required by many surgeons but not all. (This evaluation is crucial because an elevated stress profile is a better predictor of surgical outcome than the actual physical issue.)

There are several problems with this approach:

- Pain is affected by many factors, which have already been discussed. All factors must be addressed simultaneously in order for treatment to be effective, which is rarely done.
- Treatment is geared toward identifying a physical source of the pain, overlooking the nervous system component entirely.
- The surgeon may not know the physical therapist well, which can lead to poor treatment (the quality of avail-

able PT varies greatly). There are no defined standards for the level or amount physical therapy recommended before deciding on surgery.

- Only a minority of physicians aggressively deal with sleep issues. This is particularly true of surgeons.
- Surgery is held up as the "final" (and best) answer. This is just not true.

Some health care centers have elegant resources that are well organized and effective. Here I am referring to the majority of situations, where excellent rehabilitative treatments are not readily available or offered.

I am not writing this chapter to be critical of any individual surgeon or group of surgeons. We are all trying our best to make good decisions for our patients based on our experience and training. However, often our surgical training has not provided us with the in-depth tools needed to recognize, prevent, and/or treat chronic pain. It is a system-wide, cultural problem. It's extremely challenging during training to learn surgical skills as well as pre-operative evaluation and post-operative care. Some time is spent on non-operative care in all residencies and fellowships, but it is not, in many programs, presented in enough detail or in an organized way.

Recently I had a resident from another program spend a week with me, watching how I deal with non-operative care. He told me that the only exposure he'd had in his training for conservative care was to write "physical therapy" on a prescription pad and send the patient on his or her way. Yet by the day he graduates he will have the ability to determine if someone has indeed "failed" conservative care. In my training, I didn't have even his meager level of exposure.

Here are some reasons why fusions for LBP are still aggressively done:

- It is what surgeons are trained to do.
- We are paid well for performing them.
  - Even in medical systems that don't financially

reward surgeons for surgery, we still tend to be aggressive about performing surgery, as, again, it's what we do.
- In my view, you cannot fault someone for being influenced by financial factors. It is an issue in every profession. Even if someone tries not be influenced by money, it's still always in the background at some level.

• Surgery is viewed as "definitive" by almost everyone, including the patient, referring physician, society, and the surgeon.
- Surgeons feel somewhat compelled to provide that definitive treatment. If it doesn't work then at least it was tried.

Patients push very hard for surgery and many have become irrational with the endless cycle of pain, lack of sleep, etc. It's very difficult to have a patient break down in your office over not being offered an operation.

I will no longer perform surgery on patients who are not willing to implement a full, structured rehab program, including those with identifiable surgical lesions.

I am stunned when I encounter a patient who has had a flawless operation for a severe structural problem with no improvement in their pain at all, a situation which I have witnessed frequently over the course of my career. In the beginning, I didn't understand that their pain was a result of the connection between anxiety, anger, and pain. But now, I know that anger really does cement in the pain circuits.

There are many surgeons who do not operate on low back pain. When informal polls are taken at national meetings, about half the surgeons will perform fusions for LBP and half will not. Both sides feel strongly about their views.

However, it's telling that when I've asked many surgeons in individual conversations and during my lectures over the years whether they would undergo a spine fusion for their own LBP, the answer is uniformly "no." I know of only two spine surgeons who have undergone the procedure.

Our surgical training is geared toward dealing with the source of the pain. We are taught to think mechanically. There are many structural spine problems that can be solved or ameliorated with surgery, and there's nothing more reward-ing than performing a technically excellent operation where the patient does well. But unfortunately that mindset is also applied to low back pain, which, as we've discussed, is usually *not* a structural problem.

I am a surgeon who has been on both sides of this fence. I spent the first eight years of my practice aggressively offer-ing fusion surgery to my LBP patients because I felt it was the correct choice. For a long time, I felt obligated to offer some-thing. It took me a few years to learn to say, "No, I cannot surgically help you out." I finally stopped doing them around 1994. Only in looking back do I see how little I knew about the pain experience during the early years of my practice.

The pressure to do fusions grows out of the fact that when a patient sees a surgeon, it's often implied that everything else that *can be done has been* done. This visit represents the "last resort." When I tell my patients no, they sometimes explode in anger because they feel I'm refusing to solve their problem. The perceived momentum of a "definitive procedure" plays a central role in many patients' minds.

Defining "Failure of Conservative Care"

Based on the principles I've learned through the DOCC program, I propose the following definition of "failure of conser-vative care":

Failure of conservative care is when the patient has ongoing pain after the central nervous system and the soft tissue compo-nents (muscles, ligaments, etc.) have been *successfully* treated with a high level of rehabilitative care.

Note that in the case of an identifiable structural injury, surgery would be a reasonable option if there's been a failure of conservative care. For non-structural pain, surgery is still not an option.

Here is an outline of my personal standard of non-operative care that should occur before a patient considers surgery:

- You should be experiencing a full restful night's sleep for three months.
  - Usually medications are required
- Effective stress management tools should be in place and functional. You are able to effectively deal with your stress. Your anxiety and frustration must be at a tolerable level.
- Physical therapy should be combined with an aggressive exercise program for at least six months.
- If there is a structural problem, the soft tissue component should still be maximally treated.
  - Some structural injuries are compelling enough to require surgery first.
- Medications should be used on a short-term basis to effectively treat the symptoms of insomnia, pain, and sometimes anxiety, allowing you to maximize your function.
- Have specific goals in place from the very beginning of treatment, not just "I want to get rid of my pain" or "I want my life back."
- Have a clear understanding of the mind/body syndrome.
- Education—you have become very educated about the issues regarding chronic pain, rehab, and outcomes of surgery.
  - You are equipped to decide, in consultation with your surgeon and primary care physician, whether to have surgery.

- You're aware of the extreme downside of failed surgery, which I call the "catastrophe index." Negative outcomes are not uncommon.

Even if you fulfill all of the above criteria, surgery should be performed only for an identifiable structural problem where the symptoms match the injury. You are the one who has to take responsibility for the criteria being met. A surgeon cannot get inside your head. We base our decisions on our own filters and what you are saying. Learn what's at stake instead of relying on anyone else to offer up this information.

A few years ago, I took care of Jeff, a psychologist in his mid-thirties who'd spontaneously developed episodic low back pain about ten years earlier. The pain would occur two to three times per year and last approximately seven to ten days. Between these episodes he was symptom-free and his lifestyle wasn't limited by pain.

After several years of on-and-off pain, Jeff went to see a surgeon and was told that he had degenerated discs and would benefit from a spine fusion. Minimal rehabilitation had been tried. He went ahead with the fusion, which did not heal. He was then experiencing more severe pain and had a second operation to repair the fusion. Although it was successfully repaired, his pain still did not diminish. He came to me because a "new procedure" had been proposed: inserting flexible rods above the fusion across the next disc space.

By this time Jeff was almost housebound with unrelenting pain, and on methadone. Methadone is a strong, long-acting narcotic, which just took the edge off of his pain. However, he was still in pain and also groggy from the narcotics. He continued to work as a psychologist part-time, but his overall quality of life was poor.

My recommendation was not to undergo further surgery. Jeff's situation was a tragedy in that, based on our conversation, I could tell that he hadn't had enough pain in the first place to

warrant any surgery. It's tricky in that the surgeon had probably heard him say, "five years of pain," and felt surgery was
a reasonable option. The patient heard that his back could be
made better. He didn't comprehend the possibility that surgical intervention might make his situation much worse. I never
heard back from him and I'm guessing he had yet another failed
procedure.

Being educated enough to make a truly informed decision is
critical. These surgeries are elective. You, and only you, should
make the final call.

Surgery and Dentistry

I frequently compare spine surgery with dentistry. Generally
a dentist can identify the structural problem in your tooth that's
causing your pain. It can be an infected root or maybe a cavity
that has gone down to the root. The chance that your dentist
can solve the problem with a filling, root canal, crown, etc. is
essentially 100%. But what if you went to your dentist with
"mouth pain" and its source could not be identified? This is also
a common occurrence. The pain might be an issue originating in
your sinuses or TMJ, or it could even be a "mind/body" symptom.
If this is the case, and your dentist goes ahead and operates on
one of your teeth anyway, it's extremely unlikely he will solve
your problem.

Flawed Studies

There have been several studies done on fusions for LBP, but
most of them share a major flaw: a high percentage of the subjects
don't participate in study follow-up and/or cannot be located at
the two-year post-surgery point that is the standard follow-up
time frame for most clinical research projects. One has to assume
that patients lost to follow-up are doing poorly. We know that
patients who have poor outcomes are generally upset and less
likely to volunteer their time years later. You also cannot assume
a good result when the result is simply not known. Taking that

into account, marginal results become unacceptable. Often problems come up after the two-year mark, such as a breakdown of the spine around the fusion. It's been shown that breakdowns occur in 30-40% of fusions within ten years. Another glitch: most studies define a successful outcome as a 25% improvement for pain and function. My bet is that if you are getting a spinal fusion, you're expecting to become almost pain free, not just 25% better. Lastly, none of the studies compared surgery to carefully planned structured rehab.

Dr. Peter Fritzell's study[1] is the one I hear most often quoted in support of using fusion for degenerated discs in the lower back. As discussed, disc degeneration is one of the most common reasons cited for performing a fusion. However, it's also a normal part of aging and not, in my experience, a valid reason for doing the procedure.

In the study, there were 222 patients in the surgical group and 72 in the non-surgical group. (The surgical group was larger because they were using the study to compare three different types of surgical procedures.)

When I reviewed the information, I noticed a problem right away. Not enough care was taken in the diagnosis phase. In the study, the decision to perform a fusion was made in part by feel: the surgeon pushed on each patient's spine to find the specific spinal segment that produced a painful response. However, no X-rays were taken during this pushing maneuver to confirm and document the surgeon's findings. An X-ray is critical in preventing the most common complication in spine surgery: operating on the wrong segment. Making the decision to do such a large surgical intervention (the fusion) without X-ray confirmation is, in my mind, highly questionable.

In the surgical group, there was a fairly impressive decrease in pain during the initial six months after surgery. However, at the two-year follow-up the pain had significantly increased. The final overall reduction in pain was about 30%. The improvement in function was 25%. Depression decreased about 20%.

The patients in the surgical group had about double the improvement in almost all parameters measured in comparison with the non-surgical group. Based on these results, researchers concluded that the data supported the use of a fusion for low back pain. However, I question the results—the statistics are skewed because of the "non-treatment" for the non-operative group. As we've established, random treatments for chronic pain are simply not effective in the long-term. I am surprised that the non-surgical group had any improvement at all, as untreated chronic pain usually worsens with time.

Incidentally, the study was largely funded by one of the spinal implant manufacturers.

One interesting note: the study's overall complication rate of 24% (50 out of 211 surgeries) reveals the serious risks of surgery. The major complications noted included deep wound infection, blood clots, and pneumonia. Eight percent (16 out of 211) required an additional unintended trip back to the operating room. Surgery should not be taken lightly.

Worth the Risk?

One of my concerns with patients who are considering surgery for low back pain is that they haven't been given a full picture of the risks involved. When a patient is offered a spinal fusion, it's typically implied to him/her that there's a 70% to 80% chance of success. In other words, they're told it's likely they'll emerge almost pain free. However, there's little consistent evidence to support that success rate.

Even if the rate were 70%, would surgery be worth the risk? Many patients say yes—they're in so much pain they feel they can't turn it down. They desperately want to think it will work. In my experience, though, most patients and many surgeons don't really comprehend how bad the aftermath of a failed spine surgery can be. This is one of the core reasons that I am writing this book.

I've had a few patients say that even if the success rate is only 10% they still want the operation. If I reverse that, though, and point out that the chance of *failure* is 90%, they think about it a little differently.

If surgery doesn't go well, it can lead to more procedures and more pain. If none of the subsequent procedures work, it can be disastrous. The "disaster factor" has to be fully understood before making the decision to undergo a fusion.

A Careful Study

The study that firmly confirmed my observations on fusions for LBP was directed by Eugene Carragee, an orthopedic spine surgeon from Stanford. In a small but meticulous study, Dr. Carragee argued that if a test called the discogram was a valid test for back pain caused by degenerated discs (non-structural pain), then the "gold standard" of a spine fusion should predictably result in pain relief for this condition.[2] He took a "degenerated disc" group and compared it to a group who had gross instability in their backs.

To review, a discogram is a test where you're given an injection directly into a disc and a physician observes your pain response. The volume and pressure of the injected liquid and dye is carefully measured. If the response is similar to your usual pain, a fusion or artificial disc is considered. The issue I have with the discogram is that it's a subjective test: it depends on both the patient's and physician's interpretations of pain, and there is also a lot of variation in technique. It has also been shown that patients under stress are more sensitive to pain and are therefore more likely to experience pain from the injection. Therefore, I don't consider it reliable for making a structural diagnosis.

Dr. Carragee had the discograms performed in a very careful manner, with every detail documented. In addition, detailed psychological tests revealed that none of the patients had significant outside life stresses. There were 32 patients in this cohort.

The other group of 34 patients had a structural issue in the form of a bone defect called a "pars defect." Each patient had at least 4 mm of abnormal motion when they bent forward and backwards under an X-ray. In our spine surgical world this is quite a significant instability. It's believed that a fusion in this situation will work the vast majority of the time. This group, like the first, was documented to have no notable life stresses.

The surgical result for the bony defect group was a 72% satisfactory outcome. In the non-structural discogram group, the surgical success rate was 27%. The study included 100% follow-up.

It was surprising to me that the structural group had only a 72% success rate; I would've expected well over 90%. That tells me that even with a structural problem, there is a significant soft tissue component. And what about the possibility of mind/body syndrome?

The low success rate in the discogram group was surprising as well; under the circumstances, I would've estimated it to be close to 50%. Carragee's attention to detail on the quality of discography was extremely high; additionally, he had done his best to screen out patients who were under a lot of stress. Nevertheless, 27% does not even approach the placebo response.

These tests were performed on patients with low stress. Given the results, do you think it's likely that a fusion could relieve LBP in someone who's has been off of work for three years and is frustrated beyond words? The answer is probably not. There is now a recent paper showing that even if you have a well-done, warranted operation in the face of chronic pain, there is a significant chance of making your pain worse. Pre-operative chronic pain is a major predictor of experiencing post-operative chronic pain.

Although Carragee's study is a small one, no other study has been conducted with nearly his amount of precision and follow-up. If a study emerges that is larger and as well done, I will look at it. If it comes to the opposite conclusion I will reconsider my whole approach to surgery for LBP. However, today that study does not exist. The studies that suggest surgery is warranted for LBP are seriously flawed not only because they don't follow patients for more than two years, but also by poor screening, low percentage of follow-up, vague selection criteria, and over-enthusiastic interpretation of the results. The data is misleading to surgeons in training. Be very careful about your decision to have surgery for back pain based on degenerative disc disease. It does not work often enough to warrant the risks.

Twenty-two Surgeries

Doug was a young twenty-five-year-old steel worker who ruptured a disc in his lower back, which caused sciatica. He had a discectomy for the sciatica but was still experiencing low back pain so severe that he couldn't return to work. His doctors couldn't locate the source of his pain, so I would consider it non-structural. After two years of physical therapy, he was still in pain and extremely frustrated, understandably. He elected to undergo a fusion.

This first fusion was the start of a long and painful two decades for Doug. There were so many complications that by the time he saw me at age forty-eight, he'd undergone nineteen operations and was on high-dose narcotics. His fusion now extended from his neck to his pelvis. He'd never returned to work.

I was able to perform a series of operations that restored Doug's posture and greatly improved his quality of life. The improvement lasted for only about a year, though. A serious wound infection occurred, which required that his spinal screws and rods be removed, leaving his spine bent back over.

The cycle continued when recently Doug had two more major operations. The procedures re-straightened his spine initially, but three weeks later he again developed a serious deep wound infection that required surgical drainage. He is now up to 28 surgeries and counting. He is more than a little discouraged.

The tragedy with Doug is that the fusion that started all his problems was likely unnecessary. Chances are that his extreme frustration sensitized his nervous system and led to much of his initial pain. Almost every patient I see who has undergone multiple failed back surgeries had the original surgery to reduce pain with no identifiable source, much like Doug's low back pain (and Jeff's, above). When a major invasive procedure is done for a vague diagnosis, it doesn't take a highly trained medical person to figure out that the potential downside can far outweigh the benefit. Even one unnecessary surgery can set you on a path that changes your life irrevocably.

Going Forward

Our current national spinal care system needs an overhaul in order to provide patients with better care. Medical schools should educate their students about chronic pain and its related issues. Surgeons should be more accountable for the long-term outcome of fusions. They should also help patients to understand the downside of a failed procedure—when I thoroughly explain the unpredictability of surgery for a vague diagnosis, patients usually opt not to go through with it. Regardless of their decision, I will no longer perform surgery if their physical issue is unclear.

With structured rehabilitation such as the DOCC program, there is no downside. Good sleep, stress reduction, and the best physical therapy will improve the outcome no matter what your individual situation. It's the best path to a smooth and long-lasting recovery.

A FINAL WORD

Part of the tragedy of chronic pain is that once you have a failed back surgery, it's actually harder to get help. The surgeons who performed the surgery are not trained or comfortable in dealing with chronic pain. Other surgeons are reluctant to get involved in managing another surgeon's failures. The non-surgeons do the best they can to improve your quality of life, but they often take on a "survival" mentality for chronic pain patients, not a proactive one.

If a surgeon offers you a way out of chronic pain with surgery, I know that it's hard not take him or her up on the offer. Pain puts you in a vulnerable position. You do want to believe in surgery.

Many patients become extremely upset if they are told that they aren't good candidates for surgery. They feel like their last hope has been taken away. I understand the frustration. It's as if you've finally reached the mountaintop and discovered you were climbing the wrong mountain.

It's much better, though, to develop your own resources for recovery instead of looking to surgery as the only answer. You'll be more open to employing these resources once you understand all the factors that brought you down into the Abyss. The DOCC program evolved from my own struggle with chronic pain as well as my observations of what's helped my patients regain control of their lives. I am continually inspired by their determination and successes.

Acknowledgments

I am incredibly grateful to be able to share with you the knowledge I gained through surviving a severe burnout. It included intense chronic pain in the form of burning in both of my feet. I would not have made it through without the support of my wife, Babs. It can most simply be said that she was able to see the best in me. When we met in 2001 I was careening into the Abyss. How she was able to ride out this phase of my life with me is a mystery.

My colleagues around Seattle have been very supportive of my efforts and I have appreciated their clear feedback and exchange of ideas. They include David Tauben, Gordon Irving, Joel Konikow, Jim Robinson, and Mark Trombold.

Howard Schubiner is a pain specialist from Detroit, MI, who was one of the keynote speakers at a seminar, "A Course on Compassion: Empathy in the Face of Chronic Pain." He taught me that what I was inadvertently treating was the Mind Body Syndrome. His concepts are expressed throughout the book.

My son Nick and his best friend Holt Haga, who are both world-class freestyle mogul skiers, have been inspirational in teaching me to deal with adversity. They have also supplied ample material for many of the stories in this book.

David Elaimy, my golf instructor and surgical performance coach, has remarkable insights into the stresses we experience under competitive conditions. I have been able to apply his wisdom to the rest of my life. Many of my ideas are a result of our extensive conversations.

My stepdaughter Jaz has truly been an inspiration. She has come through the teen years with flying colors while experiencing her own set of stresses. She has been also very clear in her feedback about the principles outlined in this book.

It was also through Jaz that our family was introduced to the Hyde school, which was founded by Joey Gauld. Hyde is based on the concept that character development was the most important focus of education. Joey has been a remarkable inspiration and showed me that it is important to follow the path of who you truly are.

At the age of 80, Joey Gauld went through the Hoffman Process during Jaz's senior year. As a result, my wife, my son, and I also went through the Process. I was not prepared for any of the changes that occurred during those eights days. A special thanks to my Hoffman teachers, Kani Comstock, Barbara Comstock, and Raz Ingrazci. Through them, I learned that I cannot change anyone except myself.

Ron Rifkin is the designer who has contributed many hours to the design of the website and the cover of this book. He is also Jaz's father and we have become great friends. He and his colleague, Barbara Deutsch are responsible for the book's title.

I also want to thank Marty and Marilyn Chattman who have invited us into their home in the Dominican Republic. Over half of this book was written during the weeks down there when I was able to get truly relaxed.

Anne Cole Norman has been an excellent editor who has greatly clarified the flow of the material. Her persistence and attention to detail have been major factors in getting this project completed. Thank you also to Chris Kochansky who helped out with the final edits.

I finally want to thank my patients who have inspired me with their determination to get their lives back. Given the slightest chance, they have fought through indescribable circumstances back to health. This is the fuel that pushes me forward. I am grateful that I have been able to be the catalyst that has started the healing process.

Notes

Chapter 1

1. Nachemson, A. "Advances in low-back pain." Clinical Orthopedics and Clinical Research (1985); 200: 266-278.
2. Weinstein, James N.; P. Collalto; and T. Lehmann. "Long-Term Follow-up of Nonoperatively Treated Thoracolumbar Spine Fractures." Journal of Orthopedic Trauma (1987); 1: 152-159.
3. Sarno, John, *Mind Over Back Pain*. Berkley, 1999.
4. Schubiner, Howard. *Unlearn Your Pain*. Mind Body Publishing, 2010.
5. Derbyshire, S.W.G., et al. "Cerebral activation during hypnotically induced and imagined pain." Neuroimage (2004); 23: 392-401.
6. Kross, E., et al. "Social Shares Somatosensory Representation with Physical Pain." PNAS (2011); 108: 6270-6275.
7. Giesecke, T., et al. "Evidence of Augmented Central Pain Processing in Idiopathic Chronic Low Back Pain." Arthritis and Rheumatism (2004); 50: 613-623.
8. Gallagher, P.; D. Allen; and M. Maclachlan. "Phantom Limb Pain and RLP." Disability and Rehabilitation (2001); 23: 522-530.
9. Duruisseau, S. and K. Schunke. Medical Board of California Newsletter (2007); 104: 1, 11, 17.
10. Schernhammer, E. New England Journal of Medicine (2005); 352: 2473-2476.
11. Schernhammer, E. American Journal of Psychiatry (2004); 161: 2295-2302.
12. Wegener, D.M., et al. "Paradoxical effects of thought suppression." Journal of Personality and Social Psychology (1987); 53: 5-13.

13. Smith, M.T., et al. "Individual variation in rapid eye movement sleep is associated with pain perception in healthy women: preliminary data." Sleep (2005); 28: 809-812.

14. Burns, David. *Feeling Good.* Avon Books, 1999.

Chapter 2

1. Hossain, Jamil, and C.M. Shapiro. "The Prevalence, Cost Implications, and Management of Sleep Disorders: An Overview." Sleep and Breathing (2002); 6: 85-102.

2. Van der Heijden, Kristiaan B., et al. "Sleep hygiene and actigraphically evaluated sleep characteristics in children with ADHD and chronic sleep onset insomnia." Journal of Sleep Research (2006); 15, 55-62. Retrieved on 2008-06-22.

3. Dement, William C., and Christopher Vaughan. *The Promise of Sleep.* Dell Publishing, 2000.

4. Liang, Deyoung, et al. "Chronic morphine administration enhances nociceptive sensitivity and local cytokine production after incision." (2008); Molecular Pain 4:7.

5. Drendel, A., et al. "A randomized clinical trial of ibuprofen versus acetaminophen and codeine in pediatric arm fractures." Annals of Emergency Medicine (2009); Oct: 533-60.

6. Eisenberger, Naomi, et al. "Does rejection hurt? An fMRI study of social exclusion." Science (2003); 302: 290-293.

7. Winston, Stephanie. *The Organized Executive.* Warner Books, 1985.

8. Allen, David. *Getting Things Done.* Penguin Books, 2001.

Chapter 3

1. Giesecke, T., et al. "Evidence of Augmented Central Pain Processing in Idiopathic Chronic Low Back Pain." Arthritis and Rheumatism (2004); 50: 613-623.

2. Frankel, Viktor. *Man's Search for Meaning.* Washington Square Press, 1959, 1962, 1984.

Chapter 4

1. Burns, David. *Feeling Good.* Avon Books, 1999.
2. Glasser, William. *The Choice Theory: A New Psychology of Personal Freedom.* HarperCollins, 1998.
3. Kjelsas, Einar; C. Bjornstrom; and K.G. Gotestam. "Prevalence of Eating Disorders in Female and Male Adolescents (14-15 years)." Eating Behaviors (2004); 5, 13-25.
4. Laurence, Tim. *The Hoffman Process.* Random House, 2004.

Chapter 5

1. Frankel, Victor. *Man's Search for Meaning.* Washington Square Press, 1959.
2. Laurence, Tim. *The Hoffman Process.* Random House, 2004.
3. Laurence, Tim. *The Hoffman Process.* Random House, 2004
4. Burns, David. *Feeling Good.* Avon Books, 1999.
5. Donovan, J.L. and D.R. Blake. "Patient Non-compliance: Deviance or Reasoned Decision-Making?" Social Science and Medicine (1994); 34:507-513.
6. Fritzell, Peter; O. Hägg; P. Wessberg; and A. Nordwall. Swedish Lumbar Spine Study Group. "Lumbar Fusion versus Non-surgical Treatment for LBP." Spine (2001); 26: 2521-2532.

Chapter 6

1. Carragee, Eugene J.; T. Lincoln; V.S. Parmar; and T. Alamin. "A Gold Standard Evaluation of the 'Discogenic Pain' Diagnosis as Determined by Provocative Discography." Spine (2006) 31:2115-2123.
2. Beecher, H. K. "The powerful placebo". Journal of the American Medical Association (1955); 159:1602–1606.

Chapter 7

1. Coyle, Daniel. *The Talent Code.* Bantam, 2009.
2. Seminowicz, David A., et al. "Effective Treatment of Chronic Low Back Pain in Humans Reverses Abnormal

Brain Anatomy and Function." The Journal of Neuroscience (2011); 31: 7540-7550.

3. Burns, David. *Feeling Good*. Avon Books, 1999.
4. Sheikh, Anees A. (ed.). *Imagery: Current Theory, Research, and Application*. John Wiley and Sons, 1983.
5. Schubiner, Howard. *Unlearn Your Pain*. Mind Body Publishing, 2010.
6. Brand, Paul. *Pain: The Gift That Nobody Wants*. Harper Collins, 1993.

Chapter 8
1. Burns, David. *Feeling Good*. Avon Books, 1999.
2. Evans, Patricia. *Verbal Abuse Survivors Speak Out*. Adams Media Corporation, 1993.

Chapter 9
1. Gokhale, Esther. *Eight Steps to a Pain-Free Back*. Pendo Publishing, 2008.
2. H. van Mier, L. W. Tempel, J. S. Perlmutter, M. E. Raichle, and S. E. Petersen. "Changes in Brain Activity During Motor Learning: Measured With PET: Effects of Hand of Performance and Practice." Journal of Neurophysiology (1998); 80: 2177-2199.
3. Coyle, Daniel. *The Talent Code*. Bantam, 2009.
4. Wegner, Daniel. "The Seed of Our Undoing." Psychological Science Agenda (1999); Jan/Feb, 10-11.
5. Luskin, Dr. Fred. *Forgive for Good*. HarperOne, 2003.
6. Lebell, Sharon, interpreter. *The Art of Living: Epictetus, A New Interpretation*. HarperOne, 1995.
7. Allen, David. *Getting Things Done*. Viking, 2001.
8. Gordon, Thomas. *Parent Effectiveness Training*. Three Rivers, 2000.
9. Armstrong, Karen. *Twelve Steps to a Compassionate Life*. Knopf, 2010.

Chapter 10

1. Lucas, D., and B. Bresler. "Stability of the Ligamentous Spine." Biomechanics Lab Report 40, San Francisco: University of California, 1961.
2. Panjabi, M., et al. "Spinal Stability and Intersegmental Muscle Forces." Spine (1989); 14: 194-200.
3. *The Perrier Study: Fitness in America.* Perrier-Great Waters of France, Inc., New York, 1979.

Chapter 11

1. Fritzell, P., O. Hägg, D. Jonsson, et al. "Cost-effectiveness of lumbar fusion and nonsurgical treatment for chronic low back pain in the Swedish Lumbar Spine Study: a multicenter, randomized, controlled trial from the Swedish Lumbar Spine Study Group." Spine (2001); 26: 2521-2534.
2. Carragee, E., et al. "A Gold Standard Evaluation of the 'Discogenic Pain' Diagnosis as Determined by Provocative Discography." Spine (2006); 31: 2115-2123.
3. Perkins, F., and H. Kehlet. "Chronic Pain as an Outcome of Surgery: A Review of Predictive Factors." Anesthesiology (2000); 93: 1123-1133.

Recommended Reading

STRONGLY RECOMMENDED

The Talent Code: Greatness Isn't Born. It's Grown. Here's How. by Daniel Coyle

Feeling Good: The New Mood Therapy by David Burns, MD

Forgive For Good: A Proven Prescription for Health and Happiness by Dr. Fred Luskin

Getting Things Done: The Art of Stress-Free Productivity by David Allen

Unlearn Your Pain by Howard Schubiner, MD, with Michael Betzold

Parent Effectiveness Training: The Proven Program for Raising Responsible Children by Thomas Gordon, MD

The Art of Living: The Classical Manual on Virtue, Happiness, and Effectiveness by Epictetus (modern translation by Sharon Lebell)

Verbal Abuse: Survivors Speak Out by Patricia Evans

Journey Into Love: Ten Steps to Wholeness by Kani Comstock

12 Steps to a Compassionate Life by Karen Armstrong

8 Steps to a Pain-Free Back: Natural Posture Solutions for Pain in the Back, Neck, Shoulder, Hip, Knee, and Foot (Remember When It Didn't Hurt) by Esther Gokhale

Books of Interest

Man's Search for Meaning by Viktor Frankl, MD, Ph.D

Pain: The Gift that Nobody Wants by Paul Brand, MD

The Pain Chronicles: Cures, Myths, Mysteries, Prayers, Diaries, Brain Scans, Healing, and the Science of Suffering by Melanie Thernstrom

Websites

www.back-in-control.com

Helpful Organizations

Hyde Schools

Hyde Schools is a network of public and boarding schools and programs known widely for its successful and unique approach to helping students develop character. Parental involvement is a key factor in why Hyde is lauded as one of the premiere character-building schools in the world. Many of the concepts presented in this book were learned from my experience with my daughter while attending Hyde. Hyde represents the next step in the evolution of education in this country.

Hoffman Institute

The Hoffman Quadrinity Process is based on the principle that the persistent negative behaviors, moods, and attitudes we experience as adults have their roots in the experiences and conditioning of childhood. Until this original pain from childhood is resolved, it continues to dominate our adult lives (thoughts, emotions, and actions) whether we are aware of it or not. The Hoffman Process is designed to heal and transform these negative, self-defeating patterns and bring about a powerful realignment and integration of the four fundamental dimensions of our being: the Quadrinity of intellect, emotions, body, and spirit. The Hoffman Quadrinity Process uses a unique combination of proven techniques, including guided visualization, journaling, and cathartic work. I attended the Process in 2009. Hoffman significantly influenced the writing of this book, including giving me the tools to follow through and finish it.

Strozzi Institute

I have learned that you cannot calm your mind with your mind but you can calm down your mind with your body. Richard Strozzi-Heckler, Ph.D is a remarkable psychologist who utilizes a mind body approach in teaching leadership, including leadership in your own life and family. The Strozzi Institute is located in Petaluma, CA. It offers coaching services and trainings in leadership, organizational development, and personal mastery. He is well-versed in the martial art of aikido and brings these practice principles into his teaching. His tools are useful in both calming down your mind and also creating your vision of living your new life without pain.

5190930R00165

Made in the USA
San Bernardino, CA
28 October 2013